Inspired

NURSE
TOO

RICH BLUNI, RN

Published by:
Fire Starter Publishing
350 West Cedar Street
Suite 300
Pensacola, FL 32502
Phone: 866-354-3473
Fax: 850-332-5117
www.firestarterpublishing.com

ISBN: 978-1-6221804-6-2

Library of Congress Control Number: 2016937637

Printed in the United States of America

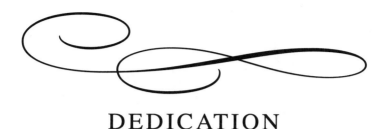

DEDICATION

To my amazing, beautiful wife, Dawn, an inspired nurse in her own right. I am truly blessed and lucky to be your husband.

To my children, Rhett, Luke, and Ava, whom I love with all I am and adore beyond words. You fill my life with a joy I never before thought possible.

To the memory of my "first best friend," David J. Hernandez. You are so loved and missed. No one made me laugh like you. Batman forever.

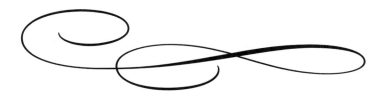

TABLE OF CONTENTS

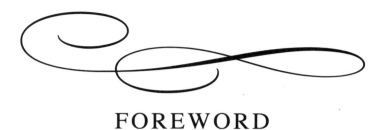

FOREWORD

I can't remember the exact date when Rich and I met. It's funny sometimes—the most important people in your life just happen to be there. You can't remember a time when you didn't know them, or exactly when you started to work together, or when a collegial relationship turned into a great, long-lasting friendship.

Logically, it must have been somewhere around 2007 or 2008, when Rich joined the Studer Group® team. I know that we were already speaking together in 2009. Again, I can't remember the exact time and place when I first heard Rich on the stage, but I do remember being blown away. He was so natural and so relatable. The audience loved him; I LOVED him.

On the stage Rich talked about gratitude and loving our work in healthcare. He told us to look for the good. These are all things I believe in as well. Rich and I thought alike and talked about the same things, although we certainly didn't deliver our messages the same way. I felt an immediate connection, and our melded ideas soon forged a friendship.

If any of you have heard Rich speak, you know that he is compassion-ate, kind, touching, charming, sweet, funny, and—of course—inspir-ing. Me, well…not so much. Funny maybe, but never sweet, and not so kind. Rich and I have often said that if we went on a speaking tour together we could borrow a title from a rock band and call it the "Heaven and Hell" tour. (Guess who would be whom?)

Anyway…Rich's book *Inspired Nurse* came out about six months before my book *Eat That Cookie!* And I must admit, I was not very excited about reading it. Don't get me wrong; Rich and I were al-ready on the road to our great friendship. I admired him as a fellow speaker, but honestly I doubted that I (ahem, the Hell from the above paragraph) would enjoy a book titled *Inspired Nurse*. I just thought it would be too sweet and too sappy. But I loved Rich and wanted to support him, and I knew he would do the same for me when my book came out. So I thought, *I'll read just enough chapters to get a good feel for the book and be able to send him a nice note.* I put a copy in my tote bag and started to read it on a late flight from the East Coast to the West Coast.

Once I started reading, I couldn't put *Inspired Nurse* down! I really felt like Rich was describing my personal journey as a nurse. I was trans-ported back to my days as a new grad and felt as if I were 20 years old again. I was reminded of all the great nurses I was lucky to call friends and mentors. At times, I was literally laughing out loud. I even started crying while reading some of the most touching pages. (Fortunately for me I was in a window seat and could turn my face away from my neighbor. Hell doesn't cry in public!) Most importantly, Rich's book reminded me of how lucky I was to be a nurse and how very proud I felt to be a part of the healthcare family.

What a gift! I mean really, how many times do we get to do something for ourselves? We are caregivers, right? We all know that on our list of people to take care of, we are last. Thank goodness for Rich! How wonderful that there is this beautiful soul who helps all of us reconnect with the joy of healing, soothing, and caring.

I heard a proverb once about a well. Now, if you know me, I usually get these things wrong. I mix them up, or tell only half of the story, so if you know this one better than me, please forgive me. But as I remember it, it goes like this: If you are the well into which everyone dips their ladles in order to drink, you need to make sure that the water gets replenished. Otherwise, when someone really needs some water, they might just pull up a scoop full of dirt and dust.

I do know that as caregivers we sometimes become empty wells. As Rich talks about in this book, we see darkness, we care for our patients, we are our own family's caregivers, and we never get to shut off or stop being nurses. For all of these reasons, we need to replenish our inner wells. We need to fill ourselves back up so we can continue to give.

Rich's inspiration is by far the best way to recharge, renew, and revitalize our love for nursing. He restores our pride in this wonderful profession. When I travel the country speaking and working with caregivers, I find that although we do great work in healthcare, most people working today don't feel great about their jobs. I believe one of the biggest crises our field faces is that the people working in it no longer feel heroic.

You deserve to feel great about your work! C'mon, read *Inspired Nurse Too*, then read it again… then give it to a friend…then get it back…

and read it again! I mean it. It is a wonderful book with great stories filled with encouragement and enthusiasm, pride and sympathy, and yes, of course, inspiration.

I am so proud to call Rich one of my closest and dearest friends, and I know when you read this book you will understand why Rich Bluni is truly Nursing's Best Friend.

—Liz Jazwiec, RN

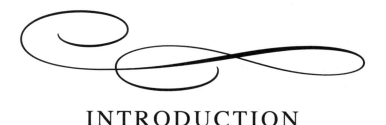

INTRODUCTION

"Nurses don't want to read books about inspiration. They're too busy. They mostly read clinical stuff," said the well-meaning literary advisor when I proposed my first book, *Inspired Nurse*. While I respected the advisor's opinion, I knew otherwise. I wanted to write *Inspired Nurse* and I truly believed in my heart there was an audience for it.

Luckily, so did Studer Group®. I'm so grateful that they took a leap of faith with me and my book. Now many, many copies later, *Inspired Nurse* has been read by hundreds of thousands of people—nurses and non-nurses alike! That was 2009. Since then I have been speaking full-time at hundreds of engagements every year, all over North America. I love what I do.

During all of the healthcare conferences and hospital events I attend, I get to meet a lot of nurses from, well, everywhere. New York, Florida, Utah, New Jersey, Texas, California, Hawaii, Wisconsin, Iowa, Toronto…the list goes on and on. (In fact, I've spoken in every U.S. state except for Alaska and many areas of Canada as well.)

Especially when I do book signings, I keep hearing over and over, "When are you going to write another book for nurses?" I had written *Oh No…Not More of That Fluffy Stuff!* after *Inspired Nurse*, but it was geared to a more general audience. And you know us nurses: We like our own stuff! I had to laugh a time or two. Now, instead of having people telling me, "Nurses don't want inspiration," I was hearing—from my fellow nurses—"We want more inspiration!"

So here it is. I listened. I wrote this book because a lot of you asked me to and I love you. (I really do!) I also wrote this book because I had a few more things to say on the subject of inspiration.

I love being a nurse, and I know how tough it can be to keep that "fire" burning. Like you, I have been through some crazy moments during my career, and over the years I've learned a few things. They helped me find my way again after I'd lost it. They helped me stay connected to hope, positivity, and the reasons why I became a nurse in the first place. Maybe the lessons I learned will help you, too.

Many great thinkers and philosophers talk about the power of shared stories. As you know, we nurses have amazing stories! So what you hold in your hands are some of my stories and the lessons I have learned from them. Some are funny. Some are sad. Some are about love, or loss, or both. That's exactly what a nursing career (heck, a nursing shift sometimes!) looks like. It's my journey. It's your journey. It's the journey all nurses take. After each story I have suggested some things to think about and some things to do, all of which I hope you can use to reconnect to your inspiration today, tomorrow, or whenever you need a boost.

I hope the journey you are about to undertake makes you laugh. I hope it makes you cry. I hope it makes you remember, and I hope it makes you think. Mostly, I hope that at the end of this journey, you feel more inspired.

CHAPTER

THE LITTLE THINGS

My speaking career means that I'm often on the road for long stretches. Not too long ago, I was returning home late on a Friday after traveling to five cities in five days. Now don't get me wrong—I love what I do. Inspiring and motivating others, from huge audiences to small groups, is my passion.

That said, unless you're Beyoncé and have your own luxury jet, traveling isn't always as glamorous as it sounds. Squeezing into seats that seem to be designed by the same person who designed my kindergarten-aged son's desk chair, delayed flights, missed connections, no sleep, loud hotels, and bad weather would be bad enough. But then sometimes, there are intoxicated seat mates who want to talk endlessly about their UTI/divorce/struggle with halitosis/not being able to smoke on planes anymore/probation officer having an attitude.

Actually that was a *real-life* conversation, and it was *one person* who discussed all of the above. He declined my multiple offers for a mint so I eventually pretended to fall asleep. However, he continued to drink and talk…to me…while I pretended to sleep. Eventually he became violently ill all over the head of the person sitting in front of him, who then put him in a headlock. Another passenger and I had to break up the fight, which resulted in all of us having at least some vomit on ourselves. I know…sexy, huh? (Some of you are thinking, *Sounds like the ER on a Tuesday!*) Like I said, travel ain't glamorous!

Anyway, my point is, I was a little worn out from a crazy week and was *really* missing my wife and family. Before the last leg of my journey, I called my wife to let her know that my flight was delayed and that I wouldn't be walking in the door until after midnight. With a four-year-old son keeping her busy, sleep was a precious commodity for Dawn, and she usually went to bed early. So I was surprised when she said, "I want to wait up for you. I've really missed you this week. And, well, let's just say I have a little surprise for you tonight!"

Was it me, or did her voice sound a little more sultry than usual? Now I *really* couldn't wait to get back. I even listened to Pharrell's "Happy" on repeat during that final flight! Soon, I was back on home turf. I'd been driving and flying since early morning, so I wanted to freshen up a bit before receiving my "surprise." I beelined for the airport men's room.

In the middle of my "personal upkeep and beautification," I noticed a gentleman wearing a travel-wrinkled suit standing next to me at the sink. As I spritzed myself with some fancy-Italian-designer-named fragrance, he looked at me as if to say, "Cologne, really?" I just smiled at this total stranger and said, "I've been on the road for a week. My wife said she really misses me, wants to wait up, and has a surprise for me when I get home!" He looked at me for a few seconds as my words sunk in. He didn't say a word—just lifted his hand to give me a high five.

Having finally tired of Pharrell's "Happy," I tuned into the love jams satellite station on my drive home. Luther Vandross, Marvin Gaye, all the good stuff. In no time, I was pulling up to The Love Shack—I mean, my house. The first thing I noticed when I walked in was the sweet smell of cinnamon. Was it incense? Some new aromatherapy candles? *Wow, she's going all out.*

And there was my beautiful wife…wearing her robe. Not the really cute one I bought her for Valentine's Day. You know, the red silky one with the black lace. No. Not that one. The other one. You know which one. Instead of Frederick's of Hollywood, I was seeing more JC of Penney. I was a little confused, but, well, whatever. No problem here. She's gorgeous! She makes velour look like silk. Plus, I was in work clothes, so who was I to judge?

At this point, Dawn kind of sashayed over to me and gave me a long hug and a longer kiss. I know it was especially good for her, as I had not only brushed the heck out of my teeth at the airport, but had also eaten an entire bag of Skittles on the way home. She was tasting the rainbow! "I missed you…A LOT," she purred.

"I missed you, too," I managed to sputter.

"Ready for your surprise?" she asked demurely.

"Uh…yeah," I responded, feeling dizzy. (Yes, I was that psyched—but in retrospect, some of my dizziness also could've been attributed to the sugar crash from the recently consumed bag of Skittles.)

Dawn stepped back and said, "Open the oven."

"What?" I was confused.

She repeated, "Open the oven." So I did, and quickly saw where the cinnamon smell was coming from. *Oh…snacks…cool!* "Well, what's in the oven?" Dawn prompted.

"Cinnamon rolls?"

She laughed. "No, what's in the oven?"

Looking again, I guessed, "Uh, pecan rolls?"

Dawn looked exasperated. "Okay, honey, this is your surprise, so pay attention. What's…in…the…oven?"

I'm thinking, *Great, what are we playing, Words with Friends?* I think I said something like, "Babe, I don't know. Toaster strudel?" I was beginning to wonder if I had wasted a tube of toothpaste and a bag of Skittles. I was expecting *Fifty Shades of Grey*, and this was looking more and more like *Every Day with Rachael Ray*. On top of that, it was close to 1:00 a.m., and my brain was not its usual ninja-quick self. "Honey I don't get it. I'm sorry."

With a sigh, Dawn said, "Okay, where do you love to get cinnamon rolls from?"

I thought for a second and then I said, "Uh…Cinnabon!"

She said, "Okay, so go slow with that in mind. What's in the oven?"

I replied, "Cinnabon?"

Dawn said, "You're getting warmer. Now say that's what's in the oven out loud."

I obeyed. "Okay, Cinnabon in the oven."

She said, "Say it again."

So I said it again: "Cinnabon in the oven."

She said, "Again! Say it three times in a row real fast!"

So I said: "Cinnabon in the oven, Cinnabon in the oven, Cinnabon in the oven. Cinna…BUN IN THE OVEN?"

I stood there stunned for a second. Dawn looked at me and said, "Surprise! We have a bun in the oven!"

So on November 29, 2013, at 1:18 a.m., I learned that my surprise was that we had a bun in the oven, our daughter, Ava! It took me a few minutes to clear my head. Dawn and I both hugged and cried, and I think I ate all six of the cinnamon rolls, I mean buns, by myself.

On July 9, 2014, we welcomed our cinnamon bun Miss Ava Bluni into the world—and it has never been the same since. She certainly was (and is) a "little thing." I started to think to myself, during many of those late nights of no sleep and trying to soothe this tiny newborn, that "the little things" can really make quite an impact. Isn't it amazing how such a small thing can have so much power? Power to make you laugh. To make you cry. To make you feel love in ways you never imagined!

Many of us assume that our "big choices" and "big decisions" contribute most to our successes in life. We often believe that where we live or go to school, if we marry or who we marry, or where we decide to work make us who we are. They do. And they don't. What I mean is, when we exclusively focus on only the "big things," we fail to see that we are jumping the gun. I think it is more true that the little choices, plans, and steps we take in any given moment are really the fuel of our success. Think about it:

- How often has a happenstance, off-the-cuff conversation—one you never saw coming—completely changed your life?
- Looking back on your life, can you recall small moments and decisions that might have saved your life?
- Have you ever noticed that who you spend time with or who you have lunch with can have a huge impact on your attitude or outlook?
- Did you ever spend literally months in school working on a project, a BIG project, and now years later can barely recall what it was about or even what you learned? Yet, can you recall a short book you just happened to come across (maybe you read it in a single day!) that caused your mind and eyes to open to things that forever changed you?

Like I said, little things can be powerful. (Like Ava's lungs at 3:00 a.m.!)

Think about the old adage "A journey of a thousand miles begins with one small step." You can look at the map before you embark on a trip and easily dismiss the squiggly line between Point A and Point B. After all, your destination is really what traveling is all about, right?

But it isn't. Each individual step along the way, from the first to the last, makes your journey what it is.

When we focus solely on the final destination and the great distance still ahead of us, we lose the ability to appreciate the present moment and have a meaningful impact within it. We also fail to consider how seemingly minor decisions can set the tone for the rest of the trip.

That's also how it is in your life and in your work. It sure has been in mine. Sometimes a "great" day or a "bad" day can't be attributed to some big complicated process that went wrong. More often than not, it comes down to stuff like having gotten one more or one less hour of sleep the night before or who you went to lunch with during break—did they make you laugh or drag you down with complaints?

You can absolutely apply my "little things" theory to being inspired, too. If you want to push back against that concept, I'd challenge you with this: If you feel it is the "big things" that truly define your landscape, remember that each big thing is comprised of…wait for it…a lot of little things. The tallest brick wall is still made up of bricks. And even then, each brick is comprised of smaller compressed pebbles, stones, and grains of sand! If the composition of each brick is ignored, the quality of the brick will be lessened, and so will the strength of the structure.

Likewise, the longest and most complicated piece of music is made up of single notes, each one interweaving with the others to create a great symphony. It is not written and played all at once as some giant single noise.

A masterpiece is not painted in one giant swipe across the canvas, either. It starts with the master dipping her brush into the paint (a brush that's made up of many tiny, individual hairs) and applying that first drop of paint to the canvas. With each stroke and each change of color, the work of art is eventually born.

So that's you. You're an inspiring masterpiece. Your work and, for that matter, your life can and should be a masterpiece of the highest degree. Priceless!

But when it comes to your profession, maybe you, like me, have often felt more like a stick-figure pencil sketch rather than a museum-worthy portrait. That's okay. It's all good. The best thing about pencil sketches is they are easily erased. So let's get started.

1. **Do one little thing to pamper yourself today.** You may have noticed that we nurses put others' care ahead of our own. It's literally our job description. You may also have noticed that this "me-last" attitude tends to seep into all other areas of our lives. Even when we are off the clock, it's hard to focus on ourselves when there are so many other items on our to-do lists, and so many "big" tasks that need to be accomplished. The idea of doing even one thing for "me, myself, and I" is totally foreign.

Your mission, should you choose to accept it (and I hope you do!), is to shift your thinking toward taking better care of yourself physically, emotionally, mentally, and spiritually. As we've discussed, even small changes can have a big impact. I'm asking you to be selfish for just a "little" bit of time each day. You and all those you care for will benefit from it.

So today, do one (that's right, kids, JUST *ONE*) thing to take care of yourself. Let me give you some starting points. Today you can:

- Say one prayer.
- Meditate for one sitting of five minutes.
- Take one vitamin.
- Eat one serving of fresh organic fruit or vegetables.
- Listen to one song that makes you smile.
- Call one friend and tell them you love them.
- Order one book you've been dying to read.
- If your budget allows, buy one "little thing" that makes you smile.
- Donate to one charity online during a break.
- Sign up for one class toward your degree.
- On the way home from work, buy one treat for your significant other or dog/cat/parrot/horse and tell them how sweet you are on them. (I can personally recommend cinnamon rolls and Skittles.)

Don't read on until you've done one of these things or something similar. Seriously.

Wow! Done already? You inspired nurse, you! Okay then, let's move on.

2. Spend a little time thinking about who lifts you up and who brings you down. Think about who you spend your time with when you are not on a shift or at home with your family. Your friends, right? Or as some of us have unfortunately experienced, your "friends." You know what I mean.

Time is precious. This life is precious. Your two most valuable and special resources are your love…and your time. So who do you "spend" those two on in your world of friends? Who do you go to lunch or take a break with at work? Who do you side with in discussions or debates? Who is the Robin to your Batman? The Tigger to your Pooh? The Laverne to your Shirley, the Starsky to your Hutch? (Too much?)

Once you have that list, review your friendships. Meditate on them. Go deep inside yourself and truly analyze the relationship. Does each person support you? You them? Do they act toward others in ways that are kind and compassionate? Do they focus on the good or the bad? Do they gossip? Are they in conflict with a lot of people? Do they make you feel better about yourself? Do they forgive you when you mess up? If you ever had an argument or disagreement with them, did they let it go or hold a grudge? Are you yourself with them or do you sometimes feel like you're walking on eggshells?

I have learned from my talks with my teenage son and also through my own life experiences that we are greatly impacted and influenced by who we spend time with. If you have raised, are raising, or just act like a teenager yourself (you know who you are!), you know what I mean. Who you hang out with in any given moment is a little thing, but it can make or break you. There are people who lift us up, and there are people who bring us down. Who you walk to your car with at the end of the day, who you vent to when things are tough, who you share coffee with, or who you switch to a different weekend shift for—those seemingly "little things" can make a big impact on your attitude and well-being.

Once you have truly evaluated your "peeps," decide as a grown and intelligent person what YOU think your next steps are. We both know there are only a few potential choices: Leave the friendship as it is. Work on it. Or walk away. What is your intuition telling you? You're pretty smart, so I am 100 percent sure you know what's best.

As I write these words, I can brag that I now have some of the most amazing friends ever. But I confess, I have been fooled in the past—and I pride myself on being really good at reading people. So here's my best parting advice: As Maya Angelou once said, "When someone shows you who they are...believe them."

3. Set a little goal for yourself—then take a little step toward achieving it. What do you want to accomplish in life? What do you hope to achieve as a nurse? What are your personal and professional goals? Normally, we are supposed to think BIG in this area! "Go big or go home!" "Set big goals!" You've heard it all before—and yes, there's a lot of merit in the notion that you should never sell yourself short.

But for many people, setting big goals becomes a depressing exercise in futility. For example, they resolve to a) lose 100 pounds, b) make $100,000 a year, and c) get their PhD. But several weeks, months, or even years later, they still are eating cookies for breakfast, are working at the same job with the same pay, and haven't even applied to school. Why? Getting from where they are now to where they want to be is too darn overwhelming. These "big dreamers" have no idea how to start achieving their big goals. They've never thought about all of the little steps they'll have to take to change their lives.

That's why I'm encouraging you to stop beating yourself up over all the big goals you *haven't* achieved yet, and start setting some little goals instead. Right now I want you to list one thing, one little thing, you can do today to advance toward a goal. Want to lose weight? How about we take it three pounds at a time? Choose an apple instead of a brownie on your next break. Want to save some money? Look for ways to spend just one dollar less every day. Want to get in shape? Do a five-minute workout by walking in place, doing a few pushups, and curling yourself into a few crunches right now.

If you're reading this book alone, see if you can find someone to do this "little goal" exercise with you. Encouragement and accountability are "little" things that can make a world of difference in whether or not you succeed! If you're reading this book with a group or department, then—lucky you!—you have a support team built in.

As you start making progress toward achieving the one little goal you've chosen, you'll probably find that your overall motivation to make positive changes increases. Goals are like potato chips…you can't have just one! To use a different metaphor, consider that a forest has never been planted all at once. It began with a single acorn, which grew into a tree. That tree made more acorns, which fell to the ground and grew into more trees. Each of those trees carried on the cycle, until the "goal" of creating a forest was reached. But it started as a little thing. It always does.

Don't forget: The little things often have the most power to change your life, open your heart, and leave you inspired!

CHAPTER

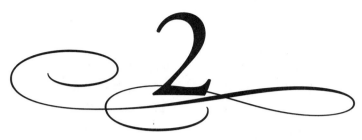

THE NEW THINGS

When you are having a baby and you already have a small child, you have to think and be smart about how you're going to "do this." Kids are somewhat territorial. (Have you ever noticed how some of their first words are "no" and "mine"?)

So when we knew we were having baby Ava, we wanted to make sure our other two kids were going to adjust well to her arrival. Now Rhett, he was fine. He's an awesome, mellow kid, and honestly, he was more than okay with his baby sister showing up in the near future. I wasn't as worried about him. And besides, at 15, he was much more concerned with passing his driver's test and being the next Eddie Van Halen on guitar.

Luke, our youngest at the time, was the one I was more concerned about. He too is an awesome kid, and at four was pretty attached to his parents, specifically his mom. Having our two boys fairly far apart saved us from the usual sibling rivalries and things that happen when kids are closer in age. Neither Luke nor Rhett had ever had to compete for "Mommy/Daddy time."

But things were about to change. My kids were about to get something "new," and we hoped everything would go smoothly. My wife and I wanted to be sure to include Luke in preparing for the baby before Ava came. He really seemed to love the attention and time we spent as a family getting ready for Ava. Luke helped us convert my office to a nursery and even had a hand in painting the new room. Pink. There seems to be a lot of pink in our house these days. Having come from a family starting with three boys, then two nephews, and then my own two sons, this girl thing was new. We were definitely breaking new ground, and that ground was pink!

Of course, I am not saying that because we were having a girl *everything* had to be pink. Not at all. But that sure is how it ended up. And I can tell you pretty much every grown woman who has walked into my daughter's room, including my 85-year-old mom, said: "I want this room!" I get it—it's pretty in *pink*—but to me it kind of looked like a tanker truck of Pepto-Bismol exploded in there. (Luke called it "the bubble gum room," to my wife's dismay.)

Anyway, my point is, Luke loved being a "big boy" and helping out. And it seemed like he was beginning to take to his new role pretty well, especially since we were making sure he was getting plenty of attention and making him a part of everything we could.

For example, a local hospital where we live has a very cute and cool class for little kids, training them to be "big brothers and big sisters." The kids learn about baby safety and all sorts of new things, and at the end they get an actual certificate! Four-year-olds love that stuff. Up until recently, if you came over to my house, Luke would insist on showing you his certificate. And if you didn't seem impressed to his satisfaction, he would let you know, in great length, all the things he learned in that class.

On top of that, we did the apparently mandatory pregnancy photo shoot. (Was this even a thing when my mom was pregnant with me?) This ritual has become as expected as prenatal vitamins and ultrasounds. But I have to tell you that secretly *I loved it*. My wife is gorgeous, and when she's pregnant, she is even more so. And of course our boys were a big part of the photo shoot, too.

My favorite photo from that day was totally unplanned. Dawn was standing on the beach as the photographer was changing lenses. At that same moment, she had some contractions and was grimacing a bit. Luke, whom we all think will have a future in healthcare because of his nurturing and loving nature, jumped up and ran toward Dawn.

Dawn explained that the baby was moving around and that it hurt. Luke insisted on talking to his sister in Mommy's belly and kissing her to calm her down. The photographer, wisely noting this cool moment, snapped the most amazing picture of Luke kissing Mommy's belly. That picture is now framed and hanging in Ava's room. Luke calls it his "portrait."

We are also very fortunate to have great friends, and whenever they would visit and thoughtfully bring us "baby on the way" stuff, they always remembered to bring Luke toys or treats as well. He racked up more Hot Wheels during Dawn's pregnancy than most kids see in a lifetime! As far as it related to our efforts in preparing Luke for the new baby, everything was going perfectly!

Until it wasn't.

One day, a few weeks before Dawn delivered Ava, I was walking through our living room and I saw Luke doing two things I'd never seen before. First, he was sitting still. That's odd for any four-year-old but especially for my super bright and energetic Luke. Second, he looked sad. And Luke is never sad.

I stopped what I was doing, walked over, and said, "Hey, buddy, are you okay? You look a little sad." Forgive me for bragging on my kid, but he's smart. This dude has been reading, literally, since he was three. No lie. He has a pretty good vocabulary as well.

He said, "I'm not really sad, Daddy. I would say I am more…concerned."

Okay. Now sometimes when he uses certain words I like to check that he actually knows what he's saying. So I said, "What does the word 'concerned' mean?"

He said, "When you are concerned that means that you have something on your mind that is bothering you that you need fixed." Good enough for me.

I asked, "What are you having concerns about?"

He looked at me, quite seriously, and said, "Daddy, when Ava is born, will I have to give up my room like you gave up your office?"

Uh-oh. I said, "Oh no, buddy. We just did that because we needed the baby's room close to our room so Mommy and I can get to her quickly at night. Your room is your room. You have nothing to worry about."

He gave me a look that I imagine the Incas gave the conquistadors when they said, "We aren't interested in your land or gold; we just want to say hi and take a few selfies in front of that really cool solid-gold pyramid!"

So even though he seemed a bit skeptical, I convinced Luke that no one would be kicking him out of his room. He seemed satisfied and we even shook on it. But I walked away realizing that even though we were trying our best to prepare Luke for this "new" thing (the soon-to-be-arriving Princess Ava who would be ruling from her very pink kingdom), we might need to dig a little deeper and try harder!

A few weeks later, Ava was born and it was a whirlwind of epic proportions. She came a little earlier than planned—my mom is convinced that Ava came so early because she couldn't wait to play in her pink palace. Did I mention there's a chandelier in there…with pink and clear crystal hearts…in a baby's room? So maybe mom is right!

Because Ava was premature, she and Dawn had to spend a few days in the hospital, and they got great care. Once the whole family was reunited, we doubled our efforts to give Luke as much attention as we could, and our friends and family did the same whenever they visited. Everything seemed to be going perfectly!

Until it wasn't.

About two weeks after Ava was born, my wife and I were feeding her in the living room. It's always funny when I say "my wife and I were feeding her" since she was breastfeeding. I am giving myself way too much credit. It's more accurate to say my wife was feeding her and I was in the vicinity, trying to make myself useful in some other way.

I could sort of see Luke in the distance, walking back and forth from his room on one side of the house to the other side of the house where the nursery is. Back and forth. Each time he closed his door. Then opened it, and came out, went to another room across the house, and did the same. My wife and I agreed that it was probably a good idea to check on what he was doing.

Now as a side note, whenever we have a child, we have a little personal tradition. We buy them a set of luggage. It's sort of our way to say, "Welcome to this world and all the journeys you'll take!" Rhett had Hot Wheels luggage, Luke got Star Wars luggage (he IS Luke Skywalker, after all!), and we bought Ava this Disney Sofia the First set. (For those of you as clueless as I was, Sofia the First is a princess and…there's this show… okay, I don't know much else but I do know we own a lot of stuff with her image on it. You're welcome, Disney.)

Why am I sharing that we buy our kids luggage? Because as I opened Luke's door, I saw Ava's Sofia the First suitcase filled with diapers and wipes and toys, being packed by her "certified big brother" Luke. I paused for a moment, taking this sight in.

As Luke would say, now I was "concerned."

I asked, "Luke, what are you doing?"

This is what he said, pretty much verbatim: "Daddy, I love baby Ava, but this has ended up being a lot more work than I realized. She's very cute when she's sleeping. That's about it. Other than that, she's always crying, and if she is sleeping, I have to be quiet, which is really hard to do sometimes when I am excited. You and Mommy are telling everyone that you never sleep, and yesterday you were so tired you told Mommy that you closed the door on the pizza delivery guy and forgot to pay him! That's stealing, Daddy!"

(Yes, that actually happened. I opened the door, took the pizza, said thanks, and closed the door. The poor guy stood there for about 10 minutes before he rang the doorbell. He thought I was just going in to get my money, but I had actually already eaten two slices and was annoyed someone was ringing my doorbell.)

So back to Luke: "So here's my idea, Daddy. You and Mommy are both nurses and you know a lot of stuff about hospitals and babies. You tell everyone that the nurses and doctors took excellent care of Ava when she was at the hospital. I saw that big glass room, Daddy, with all the babies in it and all the nurses with them. (He called this room the "baby aquarium.") So here's my idea. I think we should pack up some stuff and bring Ava back for the weekend. Not to live there forever, just ask the nurses to take care of her for a few days. That way we can all sleep, I can be loud, and maybe we can go bowling or something. (He actually said "bowling," which was funny, because at that time, we had never before gone bowling. But it was on his five-year-old bucket list, I guess!) Not permanently, Daddy…just temporarily!"

Okay, let's be clear. My very smart son, who had only recently turned five, was so impressed with the care at the hospital that he was suggesting we pack Ava's suitcase, bring her back to the nursery, and ask the nurses if they could watch her for a weekend so we could all get some sleep, get a little loud, and maybe bowl.

Now, don't judge me, but for about 20 seconds, this actually sounded like the best idea I'd ever heard. But I'm also the guy who almost stole a pizza, so maybe I shouldn't be making any serious decisions at this point.

Reluctantly letting go of the distant dream of more than two hours of consecutive sleep, I immediately snapped back to reality and calmly said, "No, Luke, we can't take baby Ava back to the hospital, buddy." He looked disappointed. I am sure he was thinking, *I said temporarily!*

In our family we have a rule. Whenever there is an issue or disagreement, we call a family meeting—anyone can. The other rule is whoever calls a family meeting gets to sit at the head of the table and decide what snacks will be served. (Sidebar: We'd had to curb this tradition a bit—Luke saw it as a way to score some good snacks and for awhile had begun calling daily meetings. Strangely, the snacks were more often closer to Oreos and barbecue chips than grapes.)

I said to Luke, "I think we should have a family meeting." He wanted to pick the snack, so we compromised on "fruit": chocolate-covered bananas and strawberries. What? That's fruit!

Within a few minutes, we were at the table, and I had some crayons and a pad. Dawn and the baby had fallen asleep and Rhett was away, so it was just Luke and me. As I sat there with my beautiful son, I realized that Ava, who certainly fit the criteria for being a "little thing" was also now the "new thing"!

"New things" are synonymous with "change," right? We had done a good job of preparing Luke for change, but we hadn't done much to help him *embrace* change!

Anyway, Luke and I had a great meeting. We ate and laughed, and I learned a lot more than I taught. We realized that "new things" (or change) bring you unexpected gifts. All we had to do was list all of the visitors—our wonderful friends—and all of the cool toys and gifts they lovingly brought Luke.

We went over the fact that when he was four, he didn't know how to be a big brother—only a little one. But now he was not only a big brother, he had a certification too! He learned to do things he didn't know before. Also, we discussed that while he could already read and sing before Ava was born, he practiced every night while Mommy was pregnant. He would sing to her belly and read stories to Ava. We swear that's why to this day (as I write this, Ava is a little past one year old), whenever she's upset and hears Luke's voice, she almost always calms down and smiles.

So, we discovered that with new things you not only learn how to do things you never knew how to do before (like be a big brother), but you also get better at doing things you already could do (like singing and reading).

Lastly, we talked about how the new things add strength to the team. I told Luke that although Ava was really little, she would grow up to be a strong, determined, intelligent person like him, and they would always be on each other's team! I also told him that when she's older and we are playing ball together, it could be he and Ava against me instead of one on one! He loved that! So we learned that the "new things" bring you gifts, teach you new skills, help make you better at what you're doing, *and* add to the team!

As we finished up our snack, I could tell Luke was processing. He looked up at me, and for a split second as I looked into his eyes, I glimpsed into the future and saw his 30-year-old self. He seemed for a flash a lot older than his years.

He said "Daddy, okay, I am open to keeping her."

Open was a good start, I guess.

He continued, "But I have two requests."

I said, "Okay, shoot!"

He said, "First, I want to keep my room. I know you said that was a done deal, but I just want to be sure. I really like my room, I know where all my stuff is, and I don't want to move." I shook his hand and promised that as long as he wanted his room to be his, it was his.

I asked, "What else?"

He said, "I will share my Hot Wheels with Ava—she can even keep some in her room if she wants—but everyone needs to know they are mine…I will share, Daddy, but they are mine!"

Luke loves his Hot Wheels! I promised him that as long as he shared, he would retain sole ownership of his cars.

So, what Luke taught *me* was that the new things (or change) call for flexibility and negotiation. New things should never be thrown on someone's head like ice water.

We went back to his room and began unpacking the suitcase. Even though I felt we made a lot of progress, a small part of me was worried. Had Luke really accepted his little sister? Was he going to be okay? Was he embracing this "new thing"?

As I unpacked the diapers, clothes, and stuffed animals, I noticed one last thing rolling around at the bottom of the suitcase. Reaching down, I retrieved the answer to my question. Luke had packed, for his sister, his very favorite yellow Lamborghini Hot Wheels car for her "temporary" weekend away.

This wasn't just any old toy. He loved this car so much he barely let me hold it. He usually slept with it. And he packed it for his sister. Wow.

Yeah, we were going to be just fine.

Do we experience a lot of "new things" or change in nursing? Of course we do. I don't think a month goes by without some new process, device, technology, or procedure being changed completely. I look at CPR and ACLS procedures today and I barely recognize them compared to where they were just a few years ago! And there are meds that you bedside folks are using every day that I have never even heard of.

New things are a constant for us. But even though change is always happening, it doesn't mean that change—even good change!—never causes stress. I think, in order to be more inspired, it is not so much about "doing change." It is more about embracing it.

Using Luke as an example, we did a lot to "prepare" him for change. It's like that in nursing. When change is coming, we train, in-service, study, and practice. We do this probably better than most professions out there! But, even with all of that preparation, sometimes the new things make us want to pack up our pink princess bags and run away!

So how can we take the example that my little son and I experienced and make it work for us? How can we see "new things" as being "inspired things"? Easy-peezy. Let's review:

1. Identify and talk with your team about the "gifts" that come with new things. What new things have you had to deal with lately? It could be a tool, device, med, procedure, or a million other things. Either alone or with others, list what "gifts" this change has brought.

Think long and hard about how this "new thing" has improved something or helped someone. (Yes, even if it was one of those things that stress us out.) Make this a discussion point.

Post the "gifts list" where others can read it. Why not? We usually have no problem complaining about why stuff is hard or frustrating—sometimes with good reason! So would it really hurt us to try, really try, to list the gifts as well? I mean, you can totally dislike a person but acknowledge that they have good taste in shoes or that they are smart, funny, or make awesome cupcakes. So, think about a new thing and list the "gifts" it has brought.

2. Ask yourself: *How have the new things added to my team?* You can take this quite literally, as often the new thing is actually a new person! In my case, our new thing was baby Ava. In your case, your new thing might be a new coworker, leader, professor, supervisor, or peer.

We get a little hard to please as nurses when it comes to new people, don't we? Maybe not you, but I have worked in places where all my peers (and yours truly) gnashed our teeth and shook our fists at the heavens, lamenting loudly about not having enough staff.

Then suddenly new people were hired! Were we happy? I'd like to say yes, but often it was no! We then gnashed our teeth and shook our fists at the heavens, lamenting loudly that "all of these new people are too new…" I guess we wanted new-ish people. Not totally new. Maybe slightly used. Just not, like, new-new. Sound familiar? Trust me, I am not being critical of nurses. I am actually just holding up the mirror.

When I became a leader, this became even more challenging, as now I was the person who was "bringing in the new" and making everyone unhappy. I don't think this phenomenon is limited to nursing. I am sure that any group of people who work and are experiencing staff shortages—whether it is in healthcare, construction, the military, law enforcement, or sales—want more staff and then struggle during the learning curve.

So let's accept that new people bring with them a learning curve, and that in order for them to become "one of us," that entails both the "one," which is the new person, and the "us," which is, well, us, coming together somehow.

So where is the gift here? Maybe the inclusion of the new person will make the holiday schedule lighter for everyone. Maybe the new person can bring down the overtime costs to help improve the budget. Maybe the new person can eventually take calls or help with ensuring that there are actual lunch breaks rather than "drive-by eatings" as I used to call them. So talk about and list how the new things (in this case, new *people*) have actually added to the team.

3. Figure out ways to help people embrace change. As Luke brought to light, we need to also be flexible and maybe even negotiate. When new things are implemented, in addition to being informed and trained, we need to also be an active part of the how and the when. Leaders need to see the opportunity to make changes based on what the frontline folks are seeing and experiencing. And leaders and staff alike have to be flexible.

I have seen new implementations blow up on both sides. When leaders were so regimented that they implemented the new with no input or feedback, it wasted time and resources. They got no buy-in and ultimately had to walk it back. But in fairness, I have also seen staff refuse to participate in a meaningful way and sabotage something that later on proved to be truly beneficial.

Maybe it's a human nature thing, but it seems that when something is "forced" upon us in overly rigid and uncompromising ways, we revolt. As Dan Collard, my friend and colleague with Studer Group®, a Huron Healthcare solution, always says, "People don't resist their own ideas." Truly. There are always going to be new things, rules, laws, and procedures that have to be implemented. For them to be successful, we have to allow room for negotiation and flexibility. This requires a balance; too little and you have bitterness, too much and you have chaos.

Change doesn't mean everything goes away…
Change teaches us that how we choose our way…is everything!

The choices we make ultimately determine our outcomes. The way we choose to relate to the new things in our world will ensure either success or failure. Don't be afraid of the new things. The great majority of the time, they bring amazing gifts to our lives. However, whether or not we benefit from those gifts still depends on the *way* we choose. Do we choose to see the way they improve our present processes, help us innovate, and strengthen our team? Do we see the value in flexibility and negotiation as it relates to new things? If the answer is yes, then we are on the way from "understanding" new things to "embracing" them.

Don't pack up your pink princess bag and throw your arms up in surrender. Instead look for the gifts and benefits and wrap your arms around the new things.

The new things will help you to do *great* things…once you embrace them.

CHAPTER

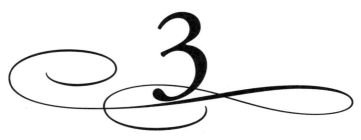

THE ONLY CURE FOR DARKNESS...
IS LIGHT

He was in our PICU for weeks, and no one visited or called. It was a mystery. His name was Benny and he was around 15 years old. He was a Down syndrome child with a significant heart disorder and had recently undergone surgery—actually, several surgeries.

The years have dulled my recollection of the specifics regarding his medical issues and procedures, but every other detail is etched in my mind. I even recall that he was in bed-space three of our PICU. When I close my eyes as I write this, I can still see him. Isn't it funny how the significant stories of our lives, especially involving our work as nurses, can be so vivid at times?

Before this particular admission, we had cared for Benny on and off. Usually a state social worker or sometimes a member of his church was with him—hardly ever family. He had a mother but I had never met her.

Benny always smiled. The sweetest smile ever. He didn't talk very much but he loved to laugh.

One day, months before this more serious admission, I was caring for him and had brought him some dinner. He couldn't choose between the two desserts I offered: Jell-O or a cookie. We were joking around and I was making him giggle because I told him whichever one he didn't want I was going to eat. I was playing like I was chomping the food, and he thought this was the funniest thing ever.

Since he couldn't choose, I offered to flip a coin. I found a penny in my locker and brought it back. This was a new concept to him. I explained how it worked and I said, "Heads the cookie, tails the Jell-O." He looked on in wonder as I flipped the coin and it landed on tails.

I said, "Benny, you gotta eat the Jell-O!" He giggled and said, "No! Both!" How could I refuse that smile? So he got both. And then he put his hand out as he chomped the cookie.

"Penny…please!"

I asked him if he liked pennies, and he nodded energetically. So I told him, "From now on, I will call you Benny Penny!" His eyes widened and he said, "Benny Penny!" He let out the biggest laugh and said it over and over again, taking the penny and placing it carefully on his table. That admission was the last time we ever got to laugh together.

This admission was different. His already-serious cardiac condition was continually complicated but now it had become much worse.

We were told that his most recent surgery had been a last ditch effort to save his life. And it seemed at times that we, Benny's nurses, were all he had. While all of the caregiving team did their amazing work, it was this group of amazing nurses I worked with who truly were there for Benny when he needed someone. None of us could ever recall meeting or seeing the mom.

It turns out that there were a few "phone calls" between his mother and the surgeons, and while there were several meetings scheduled with the full team, she never showed up. Not even once. Still, we were told that she insisted to the surgical team that "everything should be done to keep Benny alive."

Let me be clear: We didn't interpret this to mean she loved her son and wanted him by her side. While that normally *is* what you sense when a parent or family expresses a desire that their child live "no matter what," we were also aware of another disturbing scenario. This mother didn't seem to want to keep her son alive out of love. Frankly, there seemed to be no evidence that there was any love there.

It soon became clear that Benny was dying. His body was shutting down. I could tell our team was stressing. We were literally maxed on every drip.

Finally, the mom arrived for a team meeting. She stayed for only 10 minutes. She didn't want to visit or see Benny. She *did* however shed some light on why she was insisting so vehemently that Benny be kept alive. Apparently the mom received a type of public assistance, and while I wasn't privy to the details, the monthly checks were contingent upon Benny being alive.

That's right. She wanted him to live only because the moment he died, her checks would cease to arrive. She was quite clear about this fact. (While there was a lot of legal wrangling and other things going on behind the scenes, I wasn't part of that. The legal and ethics folks were busy doing their thing, and our focus, as nurses, was on caring for Benny. However, what I just shared with you is what I heard in reports and directly from others.)

I was assigned to Benny during this period, and his care was complicated. He coded several times and each time we "brought him back." His was one of the most medically and emotionally challenging cases I have ever been a part of.

At one point, after frequent visits to the OR, we weren't able to completely close his chest cavity. His organ systems were slowly shutting down. We were keeping him alive with drips and vents. It was horrible. Pretty much everyone on our team agreed this care was futile and didn't make sense.

I remember initially withholding judgment toward Benny's mother. I totally understand the ethical and medical dilemmas we face when we as healthcare people feel care is "futile." At times that feeling bumps up against a loving family's desire to give their loved one every last chance. Sometimes it's denial. Sometimes it's a simple lack of understanding or knowledge. I am sure both sides could exchange many stories about that person they knew who "wasn't going to make it" and then survived. I have even witnessed a patient who coded, was appropriately declared dead, and then while being prepped for the morgue, suddenly got back their heart rhythm. That patient not only lived, but was eventually discharged from the hospital!

Most of us are no strangers to the concept of "doing just one more thing" to save a patient's life. However, this didn't seem like that understandable situation. But, hey, at this point the mother's motives were still hearsay. Until I heard it with my own ears, I wouldn't believe it. I mean, who would keep a child alive just to collect a check? My mind could barely grasp that as a reality and my heart completely refused to. Every day I would ask myself, *Is this really about a monthly check?*

I would get my answer soon.

At work one day, about two hours into my shift, my unit secretary called and said that there was a visitor for Benny. The whole unit came to a halt. "Who is it?" I asked our secretary. In a hushed tone she answered, "It's his mom."

"Send her in."

A moment later the door opened. I met her at the door and offered my hand. She limply shook my hand but made no eye contact with me. I introduced myself and said that I was Benny's nurse. Still no eye contact. She was simply looking around. If I had to gauge her mood, I would say she looked bored. Annoyed. Distant. I asked if she wanted to see her son. She shrugged.

"Yeah, sure. Okay."

I walked her over to Benny, and she stood about a foot away from his feet with her arms crossed. I tried my best to update her as to what was going on. Just then his B/P dipped and an alarm sounded. She winced and asked, "Why is that so loud?" I asked her if she wanted to talk to him. "Yeah…" she said. Staying where she was, she said, "You hang tough now. Okay?"

Benny must have heard her because he became restless. I hoped, maybe too optimistically, that he was finding comfort in the familiar voice of his mother. She finally made eye contact with me and she said, "He smells bad."

At this point, one of our amazing PICU attending physicians was there and did a great job of gently explaining that Benny was dying. He was literally deteriorating, and it was similar to a form of decomposing as his tissues were dying. It was direct and honest but delivered with a lot of empathy. Then he talked to her about making Benny a DNR. After the attending paused, the mother looked at us and said, "You keep him alive. That's all you need to do. I got a life to live too."

If I didn't hear it with my own ears, I would not have believed it. I will be the first to admit that sometimes I talk without thinking, often because my heart works faster than my brain.

Before I knew it, I responded to her and said, "Is that all you care about? Can't you see he's suffering?" She laughed and responded, "Not as much as I have had to suffer taking care of him. Just do your job and mind your damn business." She then turned around and walked out. The doc and I just looked at each other. No words were needed.

I held Benny's hand and talked to him. We heard through one of the cardiology team members who had treated him over the years that he loved the Bible and he loved music. I picked up the Bible we had by his bed and read to him. It was a children's Bible with all of the great stories. David and Goliath, Jonah and the Whale, and Noah's Ark. The story he seemed to love most, though, was Daniel and the Lions' Den.

I have to confess that while I was certainly doing this for Benny, I may have been doing it even more for me. I was angry, and I needed to channel that energy elsewhere. So I read to him. I then turned up the music we played at his bedside, mixed a few more IV drips, and settled in for the rest of the shift. I made sure Benny was as comfortable as possible, and even after giving my report to the next nurse, I lingered with him more than usual. I drove home on autopilot, my mind still trying to absorb all that happened.

But sleep eluded me that night. I actually got up and called the nurse at 2:00 a.m. She was shocked, as apparently he had coded just prior to my calling and they were cleaning up. Benny fought on. It was probably just a coincidence, but he weighed heavily on my mind and heart all night.

The next day I was assigned to Benny again. Nothing had changed.

At another bed-space, a family was visiting their child. Their family pastor was there as well. I had caught up on my work with Benny and was now reading to him from the Bible. He always calmed down when we read to him. I couldn't help but hope that this was because someone in his life did this for him at some point. Knowing what I knew, I held on to the hope that love had somehow been a part of Benny's life.

The pastor visiting the other bed-space made eye contact with me and respectfully approached. "That's my favorite book!" he said, smiling broadly and pointing at the worn Bible in my hands. We both laughed. "I would hope so, Pastor!" He asked me if he could pray for Benny. "Of course," I responded. He grabbed my hand and began to speak.

A few other staff came over spontaneously. It was as if we had all unconsciously been waiting for this moment; there was some silent craving within us for "Spirit," for peace, for something to help us grasp what we were feeling. All of us from different or no religions, just holding hands and praying.

I began to cry. I wish it was a subtle cry, but it wasn't. If you've ever met me or heard me speak, you know I don't do subtle! I was trying to keep it together but I couldn't. Have you ever "ugly cried"? Yeah. That was me.

A few of the staff also started to shed tears. We were crying for a lot of reasons: for Benny's suffering, for the coldness of his mom, for our powerlessness, for all of the children we cared for that we just couldn't fix. For the ones who suffered. For the ones we lost.

The pastor wisely sensed this was a tough situation. He paused his prayer and looked at me. "You are angry, aren't you?" I croaked out, "More than I have ever been." I went on, "We are struggling. We are not helping this boy. This is killing us. There is so much darkness here."

When I said those words, a few of the other nurses repeated the word to themselves—"darkness"—as if that word summarized this whole thing. All of it. Just darkness.

The pastor looked at us all, and at this point, the crowd had doubled in size. This became an unplanned gathering. It suddenly felt very therapeutic and as if it were all meant to be. We all have had those moments before and know them when they happen. They are like manna from heaven, like that unexpected double rainbow. Those moments, at times, can feel like miracles.

The pastor was quiet. The word "darkness" seemed to still him. Like we suddenly spoke a language he understood but rarely heard. It felt to me like he looked everyone in the eye and thus into their souls. He nodded and repeated the word "darkness." It was as if he suddenly had the answer to a riddle that had never been solved.

He addressed us all, but looked at me as I was holding his hand tightly. I felt like I would drown if I let go. Holding this complete stranger's hand was my lifeline. He must've sensed that.

He almost whispered his questions, "Do you all believe in curing? Do you agree that for some things, there is a cure?"

"Yes," we said. Heads nodded all around.

"Well then, I ask you all: What is the cure for darkness?"

We were quiet. He smiled.

"It's not a trick question," he said. "What gets rid of the darkness?"

One of the nurses spoke the word we all knew to be true, "Light."

He nodded. "The darkest darkness on the darkest night needs only to be exposed to one glimmer of a star, one peek of the moon from behind a cloud, or one single candle, and wherever that light touches… the darkness is no more. It is banished. As long as a light shines on a place of darkness, that darkness is no more.

"It seems like much of whatever is going on is out of your control," the pastor added. "But you speak of darkness. The cure for darkness both in the literal and the 'spiritual' sense is always light."

He went on with his sermon at bed-space three. "In my faith, we call that light 'God.' If you believe, then so it is. If not, just call it love. I can tell you, the two are the same. And if you add more of the same to the same, then that's what you get more of."

We looked at him a bit perplexed. He paused and then walked to a sink, grabbing a nearby cup. He added water to the cup and then said, "Water." Then he added more water to the cup.

"I added more of the same to the same," he explained. "Adding water to water can't give you dirt or aluminum. It gives you more water. That's exactly how it works with darkness as well. Now, substitute 'hate' for 'darkness.' If you add more hate to hate, how can you ever get love? If you substitute darkness for anger or revenge, and you add more anger or revenge, can you ever get peace? I don't know what the story is here, but you spoke of darkness. Don't add to it—not in your deeds, not in your words, and not in your thoughts.

"You all cure disease and illness," added the pastor. "If I told you I had a pill to cure cancer, you all would knock me over to give it to your patients who have cancer. Right? So I have the pill that cures darkness: It's light. That's it. How can each of you be a light right here, right now, for this boy?"

We all were too transfixed to speak. The preacher in him came out and he raised his voice passionately, "That was a question!" We all laughed.

One physician spoke up and said, "We can tell Benny we love him."

"Yes!" said our preacher.

"We can focus on what we can do for him and not on what we can't," said a nurse.

"All right now!" said the pastor.

"We can be the peace we want for him…" I said meekly. He gave my hand a squeeze and said, "Now you're dispensing some light, brother."

He paused. "Let's pray for light…right now."

As he prayed, I felt a sudden sense of "something." As I type these words, I sense it again. I have my own personal beliefs of what that something is. Maybe you do too. Some of us just prayed the word "light," and some touched Benny and said that they loved him.

Standing there together, we were pretty diverse, Christians, Hindus, atheists, Buddhists, and Jews, but really what we were…was light. Suddenly the peace was broken as one of the nurses said aloud, "Heart rate!" Before the monitor could even register the alarm, she saw it. He was about to code. Again. Because of the many complicated issues that were at play, we had to work the code.

We did. By the book, as always. But this time it was not meant to be. Benny, this sweet boy whom we loved and cared for as our own, decided he was going to go with the light. Enough of this darkness. I couldn't blame him.

As our attending called the code, there was not a dry eye among us. We all helped to clean Benny up and prepare his body. We did it with so much love. Reverence. It is a duty we nurses do for all of our patients, and it is sacred. A nurse is usually among the first to touch us when we enter this world, and a nurse's loving touch is often the last thing we feel as we leave.

We all have those flashback moments, reminding us of those we've lost. Those memories are part of us: watching a young husband kiss his wife goodbye for the last time as she takes her last breath after her long, brave battle with cancer; a family holding hands as their grandmother passes peacefully in hospice; or a group of teenagers trying to grasp the sudden loss of their friend who is being taken off of life support after a drunk driver slammed into his car.

Sometimes those moments pass like a slide show before our eyes—out of nowhere. Sometimes as we awaken in the morning, we have those memories and we wonder, *Where did that come from? I haven't thought of them in years!*

That's how it is for me with Benny. He pops into my head sometimes. When he does, I close my eyes and touch my heart. Sometimes when I get change for a purchase and notice a shiny copper penny in my hand, I smile and whisper to myself, "Benny Penny." He's always with me.

After we had finished cleaning Benny up, a few of us gathered around. The pastor had exited as the code started, but he was outside the PICU and he asked if he could come back in.

The pastor had done some shopping. He had gone to the uniform store on campus and made a few purchases, and came up to several of us and gave us a hug and handed us each a small white flashlight—the kind we all use to do our neurological assessments or chart with in dark rooms on night shift. He didn't say a word. Just hugged us and gave us a small reminder to always carry the light with us.

Benny's mother did not come to claim his body. A distant family member did, many days later as I recall. We were told there was to be no service, and our request to know where he would be buried so we could visit or lay flowers was answered only by telling us someone would get back to us. No one did.

So one night we all went outside after our shift, to one of the shrub-lined courtyards. We found the darkest corner we could. We held hands and told Benny we loved him. One of us read the story he seemed to love the most, Daniel and the Lions' Den. We stood quietly for a moment, each lost in their own reflection of what this whole experience meant to them.

And then, in unison, we each lifted our little white flashlights to the night sky and let the light shine.

No more darkness for you, Benny Penny.

We have to deal with tough things as nurses. There's no way around that; we just do. I mean no offense to theme park companies and high-end hotel chains, but when they come into healthcare organizations and try to teach us "customer service skills," I used to roll my eyes so hard it looked like I was having a seizure. Puh-lease. The worst day at a hotel or theme park usually doesn't look like the worst day in a hospital. On a daily basis we see death, pain, suffering, and injustice.

It is easy to lose yourself in that.

It is easy to see the darkness and only the darkness.

Someone needs to be the light bearer. It is easier said than done, I promise. But while it is hard to choose to be the light in the dark, it is much harder to choose to live in the dark.

1. Figure out what "light" means to you. How do you define "light" as it relates to this story? Is it your humor? Your spirituality? Your therapeutic methods? Maybe it's all of the above. In a journal, notepad, or even on this page, write this question: "What does light look like?" Now write down your answer.

Here's what I wrote just as an example:

What does light look like?

Light shines when we laugh. When we find within ourselves that small smile that grows into a laugh. Light is knowing that everything has a season. Sadness isn't "always." It passes like winter passes into spring. It is temporary.

Light is friendship and love. Having people around who get you, who understand what you are feeling, because they feel the same. Light is knowing that their tears are yours…their smiles are yours. It is in this shared experience that we find a sense of peace.

Light is always there. Sometimes it is dim and sometimes it shines brightly. And like a fire, it can burn only as brightly as the amount of fuel or logs added to it will allow. It must be fed to burn brightly. It must be allowed to breathe, because if smothered, it will become extinguished.

Someone must choose to feed the fire. Someone must do the work of chopping down the tree and preparing the logs. Someone must lift the log and place it in the flame and ensure it catches fire.

All of this is a choice.

So what is it for you? Define what "light" is, especially as it relates to "light" at work.

2. Decide how you will let the light shine. So now you have a definition. You know what "light" means for you. Now, how do you "DO" it? What are the actions? I will use my definition as a guide, but please use your own. I want this to be a real thing for you and not just some words on a page. So from my "definition" above, there are several *points of light,* if you will:

Humor/laughter, friendship/relationship, choosing/deciding

Each of these themes can have an action. If I feel my unit/department/floor has had a lot of "darkness" lately, I can use my definition and points of light to address it.

So using each point, I have:

Humor/laughter: We can institute "Funny Fridays" where each person brings a joke or shares a funny YouTube video at work.

Friendship/Relationship: Each person picks a name of someone at work, and using an agreed upon amount ($5, $10, etc.), they bring in a small gift or snack along with a card or note telling that person what they like or admire about them.

Choosing/Deciding: This may be more of a personal or introspective "do" rather than an external action. Upon sensing the "darkness" rising at work, I can choose to use a very specific prayer, mantra, or affirmation to clear my thoughts or lift my energy. I can even say aloud to myself, "I choose to see the light and I choose to be the light in this darkness." I can do this whenever I feel the heaviness of despair or sadness at work. I understand that I cannot choose what happens around me, but I can choose to think and to react differently to it.

3. Think about what is stopping you from doing these things. Is it fear of ridicule? Or worry that people will mock you for being the "Pollyanna" of the group? List the potential roadblocks now. Write down this question either here or in a journal or notebook: "What is stopping me from sharing the light?" Write it. Read it. Own it.

4. Finally, meditate upon these questions. *Can you grow and evolve in darkness? Can you feel a sense of love and peace while you are full of sadness and despair? Can you fly ever higher when you are burdened by the heaviness of pain? Would you want someone who takes care of you, leads you, or teaches you to come from a place of darkness, despair, and pain?*

You most likely answered "no" to all of these questions.

If you do nothing at all, you will most likely continue to live in darkness. Can you be okay with that? If you had a disease and I had a miracle medicine that would cure you forever, wouldn't you take it? I hope that you would. I want you to know, now and forever, that the *forever* cure for darkness is light.

We can choose to do nothing or to do many things to let light into our lives. The good news is that even the smallest beam of light impacts darkness. If one person shines one small light, then one small patch of darkness abates. But if many people shine small lights, then you are talking some serious impact. Start today—right now—and choose to be that light.

Be the glow. Be the shine. Be that flame.

It's a funny thing about flames…they tend to spread.

CHAPTER 4

YOUR BROTHER IS GOING
TO NEED YOU

I was having a great day at work a few years ago—one of those rare days where it all felt like stuff was just falling into place. I was working at a community hospital in Palm Beach, Florida, as a risk manager, having just moved from my position as clinical manager of the Emergency Department. In this new role, I was able to put not only my clinical knowledge to work, but also sharpen my communication and critical thinking skills. Every day was a combination of a clinical puzzle: service recovery, quality and patient safety, and conflict resolution. I was rarely in my office, as I enjoyed the interaction with staff and patients.

As I said, this particular day was going pretty well. I was all caught up on my reports, I had finished rounding, and I had just resolved an issue that had dragged on for some time. So, I had that sense of relief you get when you cross something tedious off your to-do list. It looked like I would even get to have lunch. Lunch! For many of us on day shift, that meal is sometimes called a "unicorn meal"! Rare, special, mythical even! I pictured myself as Merlin the Wizard riding his unicorn to the magical hospital cafeteria where all my culinary dreams would come true!

I love lunch.

Then the phone rang.

Have you ever noticed how easily a peaceful moment can end because of a ring? It could be the ring of a phone, the ring of a ventilator alarm, monitor, or call bell. Sometimes ringing bells at work don't bring to mind the old story of another angel getting their wings. Sometimes it's more like AC/DC's *Hells Bells*.

The caller ID was not familiar but it was from Miami. Since I dealt with plenty of legal issues in my role, I thought, *Probably one of the lawyers*. I answered, assuming this would be a 10-15 minute conversation. I had already mentally started my walk to the cafeteria to quiet the grumbling in my belly.

"Is this Rich Bluni?" asked the caller in what sounded like a somewhat-excited voice.

"Yes, it is. What can I do for you?" I responded.

"My name is Javier. I am the social worker at Ryder Trauma Center at JMH. You used to work here, right? I don't know if you remember me," he said.

Quick sidebar: JMH is Jackson Memorial Hospital, a large county hospital in Miami. My dad had worked there for over 30 years as a maintenance foreman. After his death in 1990, JMH named a street after him (Jack Bluni Drive), and I was fortunate enough to go to nursing school there on a scholarship named after him. After graduating, I worked at JMH in pediatric ICU and at the level one trauma center in the trauma ICU. While I was growing into my role at the smaller community hospital, I still missed my friends at JMH. That place was home to me.

So yeah, I definitely remembered Javier. "Oh yeah, hey, Javier, what's up?" I said.

"Do you have a brother named Jack?"

My heart froze. That's the best way to describe it. Do you know that feeling? You instantly go from being perfectly normal, feeling good, heart rate 67, and B/P 110/68 to feeling as if you were turned inside out. *Shock.* In that split second my nervous system went into overdrive. The trauma center where I used to work in Miami is calling me and asking about my brother. My brother who lives in Miami.

I had never fainted before, but suddenly I felt as if I was going to. I have seen death. I have seen horrible burns, near decapitations, things from horror movies, and, usually, nothing even makes me feel queasy. But at that moment, I gripped the phone and closed my eyes with my heart beating so loudly I'm sure it registered on the Richter scale somewhere in Brazil.

"Yes, I have a brother Jack. Is he okay?" was my robotic and breathless response.

"Oh, my God, sorry. Yes, he's fine, sorry. But we have a patient here, Harvey. Is he a friend of your brother's?"

Harvey wasn't just a friend of my brother's. He was his best friend, a character like no other. I had known him since I was a kid. (My brother Jack is about 12 years older than me, but even today he looks three years younger!) Harvey owned the real estate agency where my brother had worked for years, in addition to his full-time teaching job. They were like brothers in every way.

Harvey was one of the funniest and most real people you could meet. When I say "funny," I don't mean like he was a comedian; he was one of those people who was funny without even realizing it. You know the type? They say something crazy, and everyone's laughing, and they're looking around, laughing along, but going, "Wait, what did I say that was so funny?"

He was also super bright and had a great mind for business. He was trusting and giving to a fault. He and my brother had been through a lot together. You would be hard pressed to find a better friend.

Javier continued, "There's been an accident involving Harvey and his wife. They're both here, and Harvey had given your brother's name when he arrived as a next of kin. When we heard the last name "Bluni," some of us remembered you and what with the sign outside the door—*Jack Bluni Drive*—we kind of put two and two together and assumed it was your family."

He continued, "Rich, I will get right to it. Harvey is very unstable. His wife has some serious injuries, but we think she'll be good after surgery. We wanted to call you first even before we called your brother. Rich, it looks bad. Your brother is going to need you. How fast can you get here? I want to time this so you are here before him."

My mind was spinning. I can't honestly recall if I asked for clinical details, although, knowing me, I probably did. I do remember my response: "It takes 40 minutes to get there, but I'll be there in 30!"

Javier responded with one word: "Hurry."

I told my team what I knew, and in a state both manic and zombie-like, I began the drive to the trauma center in Miami. I remember nothing of that drive itself. I-95 was a blur. All I could think was, *What am I walking into? How's Jack going to handle this? How am I going to help him through this?*

Not to be morbid in any sense, but you know how our minds work, as nurses. I knew, at the deepest core of my nursing soul, that this wasn't going to end well. I just knew, as much as I wanted to not believe it, that Harvey was not going to make it. I don't know why or how I knew; I just *knew.*

I also knew this would be one of the toughest things I would ever be a part of, but also that my experience would pale in comparison to what Jack would be dealing with. Jack, my big brother. How would I describe Jack? Jack is one of the best human beings I know. Super smart. Jack graduated high school around 16 and had his master's degree in his early 20s. Until his recent retirement, he was an elementary school special education teacher in an inner city school. He never left the classroom. That's like a nurse being a nurse for over 30 years and always remaining in the same department, at the same hospital, always at the bedside. Really cool. He's like a "unicorn teacher"—rare and amazing!

The bottom line: Jack is an amazing, gifted, and special human being. He's also someone I love and respect. He's like a surrogate dad to me. When I lost my dad at 22 years old, Jack basically filled the role of "dad" along with our oldest brother, Bob. Jack is who I called when I didn't know how to fix something (which was always). Jack walked me through buying my first house, and my second, third, and fourth. What could I ever do to help him?

I'm just the "little brother."

I arrived at the trauma center and was met by a few of my old friends. They brought me back right away, and I was met by the surgeon, the nurse, and Javier, the social worker. We all hugged and there was a long pause. Too long. I felt that faint feeling again. Deep breath, Rich, deep breath.

Javier spoke first, "Harvey's wife is sedated, and they're going to bring her to surgery." Long pause. "Rich, I am so sorry. Harvey passed just a few minutes before you got here."

Have you ever felt like you were sinking into the core of the earth… falling deeper and deeper into darkness? I wanted to sit on the floor and cry.

But then my "nurse brain" kicked in. To the non-nurse, this may sound odd. You are a human being processing not only bad news, but also bad news that is very personal to your life. However, there is a part of you that says, *You don't get to fall apart because there is a bigger picture here—you have a job to do*. Maybe that instinct and that calling are what preserve us at times.

I recall gritting my teeth and suppressing (for the moment) my emotions. "Where's Jack?" I asked.

"He's on the way," they responded.

"Does he know Harvey passed?" I asked.

"No, we thought it best to wait until you were here with him. He just knows that there's been an accident and it's serious."

My mind was racing between being "Rich, the brother and friend of Harvey" and "Rich, the nurse." "Can I see Harvey, please?" I asked.

A part of me felt guilty to see Harvey first, before Jack. But that nurse brain knew I had to allow myself to feel the pain and loss—and then put it aside so that I could support Jack. He was going to fall apart, therefore I couldn't. Not in front of him. I had to go in first.

The team brought me back. I could see Harvey's wife to my right, sedated, as the team prepped her. I went over and touched her hand, saying a silent prayer for her. They had been married only a relatively short while, and she was an absolute blessing and gift to Harvey. He had found the love of his life. She was beautiful, smart, and sweet. He was finally happy. My heart sunk. Life can be so unfair. Cruel, even.

"Take me to him, please," I said to no one in particular.

I stood at the closed curtain. I just needed a moment. I had seen hundreds of dead people at this point in my career. Unfortunately, many of them were children. It's always humbling and sad. But in all my years as a nurse, I had almost never seen someone I knew well, much less cared for and loved, in that state. Not since my dad years before.

I pulled back the curtain.

Harvey had the blanket pulled up to his chin. I pulled back the blanket briefly, as if to assess a patient, then quickly replaced it. Tidying the blanket and bed. Working. Preparing the area. For what? Would it make it any easier for Jack if the blanket was folded neatly? Of course not. It was just my attempt to "do something." I stopped. I put my hand on his head. The moment I touched him, I cried.

Have you ever had tears flow freely down your face? No sobbing, no sounds. As I cried, my thoughts raced: *Why now, when he was so happy? What would his wife have to deal with? Was he scared when they first brought him in? Did he suffer a lot of pain? When was the last time I spoke to him?*

It was a few weeks prior, at my house. I could see him standing in my kitchen, telling one of his stories, smiling, laughing. We were both laughing. At least I had one last sweet memory of that big smile of his.

Jack. Oh, God, where was Jack? As quickly as the tears flowed, they stopped. I had a job to do. I wasn't here for me. I was no longer even here for Harvey. This was about Jack. I dried my tears and kissed my fingers and touched them to Harvey's forehead.

As I left the curtained area, the team was just outside. They couldn't have been more supportive. Kudos to them for caring so much about my family that they even thought of reaching out to me to be there.

We hastily put a plan in place. We all agreed that my brother should hear it from me and not from the team. Maybe, somehow, a familiar face and voice would soften the blow. So instead of feeling like he was hit by a mountain, maybe it would feel more like a boulder. It wasn't much of an improvement. It was going to be horrible no matter what, but even a little softening of the pain was worth it.

I washed my face and tried to look calm. I knew my brother was going to be shocked to see me and would probably ascertain immediately that there was not a positive reason for my presence.

It was a few minutes but it seemed like an eternity. I wonder how many writers have used that line. There is so much truth to it. How time can drag a moment on! The perception that the universe is slowing to a crawl.

I stood in the lobby, facing the door. Each time the door opened, my heart leapt with anxiety. Looking for that familiar face. A face that resembles mine, resembles my dad's. The face of someone I loved and the face I would have to look into as I delivered news that would forever change his life. I felt dread. Pure dread.

The door opened and there was Jack. Wide-eyed, scared, and trying to orient himself. Then our eyes met. I have never asked him before, and it's been so long he may not recall, but I wonder what he saw— what his mind flashed to as he looked at me, looking at him. I could see a look of both confusion and relief—relief to see a familiar face, confusion as to why that face was staring back at him.

He moved toward me quickly, saying breathlessly, "Hey! You're here? Harvey and Sylvia have been in a car accident. The hospital called me. I got here as quickly as I could. What's going on? Are they okay? ...Wait, why are you here?"

I took a breath and touched my brother's arm. I had rehearsed what I was going to say 100 times in those minutes I awaited him. I am sure what came out was less than perfect. I knew that I needed to be direct. The experience of having to deliver bad news on literally thousands of occasions taught me to be gentle in tone but clear and succinct in words. The human brain can process only so much when handed bad news.

There's no perfect way. I don't even think there is a *good* way. I had done it before for countless strangers. But this was my big brother. I made eye contact with him, saying a silent prayer to myself for him, of course, and maybe selfishly for me. I was scared.

"Jack, Sylvia is seriously injured and in surgery, but she's going to be okay. Jack, I am so sorry, bro, I don't know how to even say this— Harvey just passed away. I am so sorry, bro."

A look of confusion and disbelief crossed Jack's face. "What do you mean? He's gone? He died? How could he be dead? What are you saying?"

"Jack, I am sorry, bro. He just passed a few minutes ago. They did all they could. I am so sorry. I am so sorry."

Right now, I can't even bring up the image of my brother's face in my mind without feeling the same way I felt in that moment: Crushed. Sick. Sad doesn't even begin to describe it. Now multiply that by 1,000, and that was how Jack felt.

We embraced. He sobbed. The next few moments are a blur. I am sure we spoke some more. I answered his questions. As always, in those moments, the brain goes into shock.

He relived the last times they spoke. He asked the same questions several times. He was overwhelmed. The situation was compounded by the fact that his wife, Julie, was away with their boys on a camping trip, and this occurred in pre-cell phone days. His normal rock and support system, his wonderful wife, was thousands of miles away and hard to reach. It was just me and Jack.

At this point, some of the team stepped in and answered a few questions. Jack and I remained with our arms around each other. After a pause, I asked him, "Do you want me to bring you to see him?" I knew he would need this closure, but I also knew how hard it was going to be. It's one thing to hear that your friend is dead. It's another thing entirely to see that your friend is dead.

Jack's answer was short. "Yes."

We walked into the trauma area, and I brought him to the curtain. I was so scared for him. I knew these next few minutes would be some of the worst of his life. *Please, God, let me say the right things or say nothing. Please help Jack.*

I may have said some words of preparation, but I don't recall them. I held Jack and pushed back the curtain.

I apologize, dear reader, as I have a complete block as to what exactly transpired. I know only that I witnessed the heartbreak of someone I loved dearly. I just held him. Silent tears fell from my eyes. I was helpless. I couldn't fix this. All I could do was hold my brother as he sobbed. That was only the second time I had seen Jack cry in my life. The first was when our dad died.

It never struck me at the moment, but two of the toughest events of Jack's life, two of his biggest losses, intersected here. His best friend Harvey died on the street named after our dad. I can't help but look back on that day and hope my dad was there with us. Maybe his spirit even embraced Harvey as he transitioned. My dad loved Harvey, and Harvey loved my dad. Just as I was a familiar face for my brother in this painful transition, maybe on some spiritual plane that none of us can even comprehend, my dad was a familiar face for Harvey. I know that my dad would have greeted him with open arms. Whether that is true or not doesn't matter. It gives me a sense of peace.

Jack and I remained there for a while. It was hard for him. My brother, the kind teacher, the sensitive, loving husband and father, was out of his element here.

I do recall that as we left Harvey, Jack hugged me and said, "Thank you for being here."

In his moment of absolute grief and pain, he was thanking me? I didn't feel as if I had done *anything*.

Many years have passed since that day. I know Jack still misses his friend. While time certainly eases the pain, it is always there for him. I can never repay my brother for all he has given to me: his love, his advice, his friendship. I love him, and that is all I can do. I only hope, in some small way, that I was able to take even 1/1,000 of his pain away.

Looking back, this incident really clarified a few things for me. First, we often can't heal our patients or stop them from hurting. We can't take away their cancer or restore their shattered limb. Instead, we measure our victories in small strides, like reducing pain from a 9 to a 6, or improving an O_2 saturation from an 85 percent to a 90 percent. If we celebrated only the "miraculous healings" we occasionally see and ignored all the "little things," we'd be in a constant state of hopelessness.

Second, you never know when your world will be shaken up, when a "bell" will ring, calling you forth to face something in your own life. You never know when you will be "called" to help someone. You never know when you will hear that knock at the door at home and open it to a frantic neighbor, holding their choking child in their arms. You never know when you'll be in a mall, hear a scream, and see people standing over an elderly man turning blue on the ground. You never know when the person who needs you will turn out to be your husband, your sister, your friend, or your brother.

And that brings me to the third thing I learned: We never "stop being nurses." We're always on. (I'd imagine it's the same for lots of caregivers: paramedics, police officers, physicians, and more.) Sure, nurses have to deal with challenges in our lives. We face illness, divorce, financial worries, and more, just like a banker or a computer programmer or a saleswoman deals with "life outside of work." But let's be honest: Even when we're confronted with personal, health, or natural disasters, what is expected of us and what we expect from ourselves is very different from our peers in other professions.

Returning to a previous example, when we walk through a mall and see someone collapse, we go to work. When a banker walks through a mall and sees someone open their wallet to pay for something, she doesn't walk over and help the other person count their money. Nurses don't get to "turn it off" the way that some other professions can.

To use a more personal example, I think about all of the hurricanes I've been through in Florida, starting with the worst I have ever seen, Hurricane Andrew. Many nurses I knew at the time lost the roofs off of their houses (or their entire house), had their cars destroyed, had their apartments blown to pieces and barely survived—and they came to work as soon as they could. Some of them were even picked up by the National Guard in Humvees to help get them there!

Were those nurses stressed? You bet! Did they wonder if their families would have a safe place to sleep, food to eat, or a school to go to? Of course. But unlike a lot of other people, they knew that if they didn't show up for work at the ICU or L&D Department, this natural disaster would claim even more lives.

(I mean no disrespect to any other jobs or professions, but I highly doubt Macy's or the local car dealership or bank would call their employees and demand they show up ASAP! "We better be ready for the 'After-Hurricane Blow-Out Sale' on Mustangs! Hurry up, people! Forget your own problems. We've got cars to sell!!!")

Heck. No. Those folks were told to stay home. But we (and, of course, our fellow caregivers of all stripes) had to come to work. And when I say "had," I don't mean we were "forced." In fact, I saw many nurses show up on their own because they felt compelled to help. We didn't stop being nurses just because we were faced with our own difficult circumstances.

I am sure the same thing happens when there is a hurricane, tornado, earthquake, or flood anywhere in the world. We patch up our lives and find that one semi-clean pair of scrubs, kiss our families on the head, and "go to work." We don't know any other way.

But while that all sounds admirable and heroic (and it is!), it also is tough. We should take a moment to acknowledge that. We make sacrifices. We put ourselves aside for the greater good. We don't walk away from a challenge, a mission, or a disaster.

Ever.

When that doorbell rings, when the phone starts blowing up, when storms rage, and when flood waters rise, somewhere there's a nurse taking a breath, closing their eyes and saying a prayer, and stuffing those extra scrubs in a backpack because they know it's about to get real.

You can never really be "prepared" for the unexpected event. Not truly. We don't leave the house thinking, *I will probably see a car flip over on the highway and land in a ditch. I better leave 30 minutes early and wear comfortable shoes so I can help rescue the passengers.* No. We all know if something like that is in the cards, it will happen when you're wearing heels or dress shoes and running 30 minutes late!

What we *can* do is reflect on the stories we have experienced, focusing on when "the bell rang." Do that, and try *not* to be inspired!

1. Write down your story about a time when you were "called" unexpectedly. That flight you took when the flight attendant suddenly ran to the front of the plane and asked over the P.A., "Is there a nurse or physician on board?" What was that like? What happened? How did you feel? What impact did you have on the event? What impact did the event have on you? This is a great exercise to do with other nurses. Do a story exchange. Call it a "When the bell rang…" exercise. If you do this as a group or a department, it is a pretty incredible exercise. You will learn a lot about yourself and your peers.

2. Journal about how you feel as "the nurse in the family/circle of friends/neighborhood." Is it fun? Stressful? Do you feel valued? Do you sometimes feel like shaking your head when for the 100th time you tell a loved one that if they keep smoking/drinking/eating sweets too much, XYZ will happen (and it does…and they're always surprised)? What does that bring up for you internally? Frustration? Anger? This is also a great exercise to do with other nurses. Why? Because sometimes it takes a nurse to understand a nurse. Discuss these times when you felt like you were not being listened to or respected by those you love or those who sought your advice.

3. If possible, talk about the "When the bell rang…" event with the people involved. Maybe a friend's child had a seizure when you were having a play date together, or you spent the night in the ED with your cousin when her husband was in a bad car crash. If it is possible, and if they are able, talk about that day with the other people involved. Have dinner with them. Have some coffee. Ask them what they saw and felt, and how they viewed your role in their life event. It's interesting to learn what it looked like to them.

I remember helping a child and her mom on the roadside after a bad crash. (I actually resuscitated the child—you can read the story in *Inspired Nurse*.) I was terrified and I was probably a nervous mess, but when I had a chance to talk to the mom days later in the hospital,

I realized she saw me in a very different way. I learned more about myself than I ever imagined just hearing her take on the event.

The bell rang and I got the call—the call we all dread. A voice said to me, "Your brother is going to need you." But ultimately, for us nurses, that call happens in many different ways. I've learned that nurses see everyone as their brothers or sisters. We *always* take that call.

It's what makes us the inspired nurses that we are.

CHAPTER

5

HAND...STAY...HELP

Being a nursing student is never easy—not a moment of it. It is the hardest thing most of us have ever done and will ever do.

Most nurses agree, looking back on school, that it prepared and empowered us, taught us, and sometimes scared the heck out of us. I would imagine nursing school ranks, in difficulty, close to Navy SEAL training. (Of course I am kidding, but once I was taking care of a former SEAL, and as he watched me make his bed, he asked if I was former military. He said he was impressed with my precision. I was too, until I bragged about this to some of my guy friends. Needless to say, most guys aren't impressed if your sheet folds are SEAL-worthy. Whatever.)

Some of our most memorable moments happened in nursing school. Many of us saw our first baby born, our first death, our first everything during this time—especially if you went to a school like mine. It's gone now, but Jackson Memorial Hospital School of Nursing had been around for a long time by the time I got there.

It was that rare breed of school in which classes *and* clinicals actually took place at a large county public hospital. We saw it all. Jackson grads were clinical ninjas by the time they graduated. My friends in other programs were sometimes envious of what I saw during my clinicals. Burns? GSWs? Head traumas? Celebrities who partied too much on South Beach and crashed their Bentleys? Check. Check. Check. Check. And that was just in the first three weeks of school!

At a certain point in your school progress (I think it was after the second year), you were allowed to work at the hospital in what was called a PCT (patient care technician) role. You pretty much became a nursing assistant. You could do baths and transports, take vital signs, and change bed linens. (The latter of which, in my case, could even impress Navy SEALs! But I should be cautious about bragging about my bed-making skills in the event my wife reads this book.) You got to rack up some experience, learn more about the areas you were interested in, and also make some money along the way—a much-needed benefit when you were in school five days a week full-time.

Back then, I wanted to be a trauma nurse. And eventually, years later, I worked in a trauma ICU. Funny thing is, when I was asked as a nursing student where I wanted to work and where I would never work, I swore that I would never work in pediatrics or ICU...and then I spent eight years in a pediatric ICU *before* moving to trauma. And I loved it!

You never know, do you?

I remember my behavioral health rotation. Like many other areas in nursing, students either loved it or hated it. I loved it. I found it interesting, challenging, and at times, overwhelming.

As a student, I got along really well with Peter, the director of the be-havioral health unit. He was a very smart up-and-coming leader. He cared about his staff and his patients, and he was one of the most wel-coming leaders toward us students. When he asked me to be a PCT in the adult unit, I felt pretty honored! I was torn between working in his department and a neuro department. But Peter was relentless, so I decided that I would give behavioral health a try.

I like to be real. As a person, a husband, a dad, a nurse, and a speaker, as I travel around North America speaking at hundreds of confer-ences. I also like to be real when I write. Even if the story is partially "fictional" to provide privacy. So I hope what comes next comes out as "real" and not "negative."

First, though, a disclaimer: When you write books with titles like *Inspired Nurse, Oh No...Not More of That Fluffy Stuff! (The Power of Engagement)*, and the one you're holding in your hand now, it's im-portant to tread carefully. You want to be positive, inspiring, motivat-ing, and uplifting. But sometimes that means you have to share the things that didn't go well. That's life. That's nursing. So, here comes the "real" part.

This particular department was a tough place to work. There were some good folks working there, but I was also learning that while nursing was 99 percent made up of caring, brilliant, and heroic people, there was also the other 1 percent hanging around the edges. These people, that other 1 percent working in various roles, were also great teachers. *Amazing* teachers, in fact. They taught me exactly what I *didn't* want to be like when I became a working nurse. Like I said, there were some truly awesome folks in this particular unit— Peter was one—but looking back I realized one of the reasons he was so aggressive about recruiting us students is because he must've had a sense that he needed some "new blood" in that somewhat-toxic department.

I remember my first shift as a PCT. I was nervous and excited. We had some intense patients there; they had very challenging psychiatric issues coupled with medical issues. As we all know, those two factors go hand in hand and make the work that our behavioral health peers do some of the most challenging and unique in healthcare. I was determined to blow everyone away. My patients were going to be clean, happy, and safe. The staff was going to love me. I was going to be the best PCT EVER! (Stop gagging…I was 23!)

So before the shift started (and this was 7:00 p.m.-7:00 a.m. so Peter and the other day shift leaders were gone), I was introduced around by the charge nurse. A few people flashed smiles my way but mostly they displayed, as they say in behavioral health, "flat affects."

Hmm. Tough crowd. The group broke up and the charge nurse pulled me aside for what I knew would be my welcoming speech, maybe a gift, or even a hug.

Yeah…no.

"Listen," he said. "We do things how we do things here. If you want to fit in, keep your head down, your mouth shut, and know your place. If not, you won't last. We don't trust outsiders. We didn't want you here. Some people think you're a spy, so watch your back. I told everyone that you were an okay kid and would take work off their hands so they're watching you. Mind your manners. Don't rock the boat and you won't get thrown overboard. Understand?"

Okay, what just happened? I thought this was my first day as a PCT; I didn't realize I was pledging for a biker gang! I was a kid at the time and very intimidated by this older man, my superior, who was also 6'4" and very intense. I think I just nodded my head.

"Good. You're a smart kid."

My first shift went by quickly although at times I found myself looking over my shoulder. Most of the team was pretty cool. I never saw a patient mistreated or neglected. Even as intimidated and young as I was, I would've reported that ASAP. It wasn't anything like that. It was more of an attitude of "don't do more than you need to."

I worked there for a few months and found my stride. During this time, I worked various shifts. Some were better than others—a lot better. Whenever I worked with the crew from my first night, I still did my work and watched and learned. My focus was on these patients.

The majority of them were homeless, mentally and medically ill—many of the very same people you might pass as they sleep on a train platform or you might see wandering the streets talking to themselves.

Despite the difficulties, I had many amazing experiences there with some of the staff and patients. I can recall many times another tech or nurse and I would take a homeless patient and give them the full "spa treatment": bath, haircut, nails trimmed, the works. It's amazing how sometimes that, more than the meds or even the therapy, did so much to change the state of a patient. Who would've thought that the "bed bath" skills I was learning in school could be so miraculous and transforming?

During one shift, they admitted an elderly man named Matheus. He was probably in his late 60s, African American, and decently groomed although disheveled and dirty. He was found wandering the Miami streets, and the police were called when he walked into a fast food restaurant and began yelling and crying. No words. Just gibberish. He was sent to us.

Unfortunately, the night he arrived, most of the same crew from my first night were on staff. Matheus was assigned to me as his PCT after they did the intake process. A resident physician quickly assessed him. Besides being assessed as "non-verbal," he was given a diagnosis of, I believe, schizophrenia or something along those lines.

But something "just wasn't right." I wonder how many nurses have started a story or phone call to an on-call physician with that line. You know the feeling. That gut feeling. All seasoned nurses have it. And apparently even some student nurses too, as I learned.

My first call of business was to get him cleaned up. I remember noticing that while his clothes were dirty, they didn't appear worn or old. Odd. Usually the homeless have very worn clothes—tears, rips, frays, in addition to being dirty from living on the streets. His clothes were certainly dirty, and maybe this sounds odd, but they seemed "newly dirty." Also, as I talked to him, he seemed very alert. It was his eyes. He looked deep into my eyes. There was not only intelligence in his eyes but also something else. Presence? Emotion? I remember also noting that he seemed physically weak to me.

Now, my "assessment vocabulary" at the time was fairly novice, but I grabbed the resident and pulled him aside and shared with him that something "just wasn't right" with Matheus. This poor exhausted resident looked at me and then looked at my PCT badge and thought better of trusting my "medical opinion." Understandable. But throughout the next few shifts, something in my gut just wouldn't let up. I shared my concern with each nurse and each doctor I encountered.

On one of those shifts, "the crew" I spoke of on my first day was on. I got pulled into the break room and was told I needed to back off. *They* were the experts. They had seen 100 patients like Matheus before. I knew nothing and I was creating a lot of drama. I was reminded to "know my place," but I knew at that point my "place" was to help Matheus.

Then I got the affirmation I needed. As I was taking care of Matheus, I found myself spending any chance I could with him. I was holding his hand and I said, "Squeeze my hand if you understand me." I had been doing this to no avail over the days since he had been admitted, and then it hit me. I was always holding his right hand. I don't know where it came from, certainly not from my "brilliant clinical acumen and bedside experience" but something inside of me told me to switch hands. I did.

Holding his left hand, I looked into those deep expressive eyes and I said, "Matheus, if you understand me, squeeze my hand." And he did.

My heart leapt. "They" were all saying he was deeply psychotic and unresponsive. I saw them assess him. But all of a sudden, I was realizing my gut was right, there was something else going on. This wasn't because I was a "clinical genius"; I was a student with very little experience, but I was also an intuitive guy who was developing that "nurse's instinct."

I grabbed both of his hands. "Matheus, squeeze." He did. But only the left side. That's why he was weak. That's why he wouldn't stand on his own. The "crew" said he was being "uncooperative."

No. He was weak on one side of his body. I made a beeline for the charge nurse. Yes, that one. I told him what I noticed. He didn't look up. "You're not as good of a listener as I thought," was all he said.

"Are you going to assess him or not?" At first he was taken aback by my forceful tone. Then he smiled. "Does it look like it?" he asked and went back to ignoring me.

But there was someone else there. Another nurse. One of the "99 percent of us," chatting with a resident physician. I must have looked really concerned, because when our eyes met, they both motioned for me to walk away from the charge nurse. They quickly followed.

When the three of us were at a safe distance, I told them everything I had seen over those few days. I also told them that if they didn't take this seriously, I was going to find the chief of the department and drag him here myself, even if it meant my job. Even if I was wrong. I could tell they were willing to listen.

I told them what I had felt. How Matheus's eyes seemed to be pleading, how he always made eye contact with me, and that whenever I left him to do anything, he got upset. I told them I was worried he was being overlooked and lumped in with "everyone else." But it wasn't until I described what had just happened with his grip that their eyes widened.

"Let's go," they said in unison as I led them to Matheus. They crowded around Matheus and me. As soon as I sat down and held his hand, he started to make noise, like he was going to scream. Something was building up.

And then words came out. Barely understandable.

He said: "Hand...stay...help."

I almost cried. The nurse and physician moved in immediately. They began what I now know was a full neuro assessment. They called the attending, and yes, they called the charge nurse as well. If looks could kill, I'd be writing this from my coffin right now. I can only imagine what he thought when he saw several residents and nurses along with lab and radiology transport dashing around. Let's just say he was clearly not thrilled with all of the extra work I had created. Oh well.

The rest you all know. What followed was a whirlwind of studies and tests. Matheus wasn't a behavioral health patient. No. As the days progressed, the team learned a lot more about him.

Matheus was a retired man who lived alone. He had apparently had a stroke, and in a moment of confusion, wandered from his house and somehow boarded a bus without paying a fare. He exited the bus, possibly removed by the driver for not paying, a few miles from his home and began wandering the streets. In his weakened state, he simply laid down when he was tired and grew more and more confused until he wandered into a fast food joint where he was picked up by the police.

Because of his disheveled appearance, he looked like all of the other confused homeless wandering the streets and found himself here.

As I recall, he was moved to a medical ICU and got great care. He made a lot of improvements and was able to go to an assisted living facility and then eventually home.

And boy, did I learn.

The next time I came to work, it was a day shift. Peter and the attending physician were waiting for me. I don't remember most of what they said except for these words: "You made a difference. You belong in nursing. Thank you."

I think I repeated that to my wife, my family, and every friend I had at the time, every day for about two years! It meant the world to me. To be affirmed. To know that this path I was on was the *right* path.

As far as "the crew" goes, I couldn't tell you what became of them. I can tell you they were not a true representation of who and what the vast majority of nurses are, but we all know they're out there. I know Peter had his hands full and I heard that over time, he made some awesome changes to that department. Rome wasn't built in a day. But it got built eventually!

After that summer, I chose to work elsewhere. A fact of life is that sometimes we learn more from the bad examples and experiences than we do from the good ones.

I used to think that you knew when a path was "right" if everything was golden. You know? If the path had flowers and butterflies flying around and the sun always shined on the path. I learned, however, that you can't always define "the right path" by the pretty flowers growing alongside. Not always. Sometimes even the right paths have some stones on them, weeds, thorns, and even boulders blocking the way. Sometimes even the "right paths" get a little dark and scary.

Maybe traveling the right path sometimes means being tested. When it gets tough and dark, what do you do? Sometimes, when you hang in there, you realize that you were always on the right path. You just needed those bumps and thorns to help you get focused.

But this whole experience taught me something even more important. Three words.

Trust. Your. Gut.

I think inspiration is a "gut" thing. I think it is much more spiritual and "heart-based" than it is intellectual or science-based. That's just me. But many times I have found myself, after making the wrong choice or decision, smacking my head and wondering, *Why didn't I trust my gut on this?!*

So many times, personally and professionally, I chose the wrong relationships, wrong friends, wrong jobs, wrong cars, wrong hair styles (when I had hair!). I look back on each instance and can remember getting a gut feeling that I should end this relationship, or that a friend seemed a little fake, but stayed in the mix—only to regret it.

Trust. Your. Gut.

1. Think about a time you truly trusted your gut. Remember the time you took an alternate route to work and learned later that there was a big accident on the road you normally travel? Or the time you checked on a patient who was totally stable, on a hunch, only to have them code moments later. What was it that turned you away from that road? What brought you to that patient at the exact moment they needed you?

2. Share your "gut instinct" stories. Get a few nurses together (maybe do this as a departmental or nursing school project) and discuss your various "gut" stories. Share them in detail. I bet if you get at least five together, you will be shocked by how often you hear a story and say, "Wait, that happened to you, too?"

3. During your next workday, commit to listening to your gut. No, not the growling sound when it's 10 minutes past lunch—the other thing! Listen to your gut in every instance. When you are admitting someone and listening to their history, what's your gut saying to you? When you walk past a patient's room and make eye contact, what did your gut just tell you? When you talk to another nurse, physician, student, or professor, what comes up for you? Maybe keep a journal of this info and actually look to see if there's a pattern. Imagine what you'll learn! Maybe you can teach those around you how to better connect to their instinct.

4. Talk to new/newer/student nurses about "trusting their gut." There are some amazing nursing school curriculums out there and some even more amazing nursing educators. And those educators have a lot of ground to cover in order to prepare our future nurses. So if you are one of them, think about discussing "trusting your gut" with your students.

Maybe you're not a nursing educator but you're around students often or get to give orientation to new nurses. Make sure you talk with these future or brand new nurses about the importance of instinct and how crucial it is to learn to trust those feelings.

A great way to have this conversation is first to ask if they have ever had a "gut instinct" either to do or not do something. Then once affirmed, ask them where they personally think that feeling comes from. Expect lots of diversity there. Some think it is God speaking to them; others think it is angelic beings. Some will tell you it is merely a coincidence, while others will tell you it comes from that mysterious 90 percent of our brain we never use. Some will even tell you it is magic.

I have my beliefs; you have yours. Maybe they're the same, maybe not. Vive la différence!

The neat stuff is in the discussion. The inspiring stuff is when you share one of your stories and someone gets goosebumps or tears up, or when someone tells their story and your eyes get wide and you feel like you're right in the middle of their story. You might even feel it *in your gut!*

It's some powerful stuff to share with others. But it is also powerful to acknowledge.

We need more "gut instinct" in nursing as much as we need more science. This work that we do encompasses more than one verifiable realm. It is physical, intellectual, mental, and spiritual.

Nursing is an "all of the above" profession...especially among the inspired. Try some of these exercises. I did. I found them incredible and borderline miraculous, actually. You may find you're more "gutsy" than you realize!

Before Matheus went to the assisted living facility, I was able to visit with him. He still had some deficits but was doing much better. His speech wasn't great, but his eyes were clear. When I walked in the room, he looked at me blankly for one second, like he wasn't really there. Then suddenly, there he was!

I walked over and sat on his bed. He grabbed my hand first. He stared into my eyes, actually more into my spirit. We sat like that for several minutes, like a long-lost father and son who were just grateful to have found each other. He didn't say a word, but he put his arm out, and we hugged each other. As we pulled away, he was still intently looking me in the eyes. And both of our eyes filled with tears.

While he didn't say a word, I still heard him. I heard him loud and clear.

"I love you too, my friend." I answered.

CHAPTER

JUST SOME DUSTY
OLD NOTEBOOKS

"Another day at the carnival," said our ED unit secretary, surveying the madness. It was another packed house, and then some, in the ED.

We were in the middle of what we called the "season" in this part of Florida: a time when the seasons are not really noted by the color changes of the trees, but more by the color changes of the license plates! See, in South Florida—specifically Palm Beach—the trees don't change color when the weather cools; the only color changes we see are the license plates that read New York, Massachusetts, New Jersey, and Pennsylvania. Our season is also noted by the type of birds that fly south for the winter. Not real birds—"snow birds."

During the winter, all the retirees from up North who have lived long enough to deserve a break from the cold come down to seasonal rentals or vacation homes to stay warm and enjoy the Florida sun. Things get crazy all over town, restaurants are full, grocery stores are packed, and, of course, hospitals are swamped.

On this day, our ED was not only full; we were maxed out and then some. Every room was packed, stretchers were in the hallways, and our "holding area" was also full to the top. I've never seen anything like it anywhere else. The hospital was also full, which meant that as patients got admitted, we kept them in the ED. So the ED nurses were also ICU nurses and med-surg nurses and CNAs. Sometimes, we kept patients for days on end. Those nurses were amazing. Still are.

As the secretary and I took one second to look across the abyss of madness that was the ED, we both sighed at exactly the same time, which made us both laugh more.

The sign of a good team is the ability to laugh even when things look tough. "We gonna get through this, Boo," she said as we both high fived.

We were the ED. We had no choice.

"Can someone transport?" Shannon, one of the most seasoned nurses, called out.

I was the ED clinical manager at the time, and I tried my hardest to be as hands-on as possible. So I called back, "I got you, Shannon," and went over to her bedspace—actually, hall space—that had a temporary curtain pulled around it to give it at least a semblance of privacy. ("Semblance" being the operative word.)

"Thanks, Rich! I need this gentleman transported to holding. At least they have beds there so I can get him off this stretcher. He's a sweet-heart. Poor man. He's been here for two days already!" she said.

"Sure, anything for you!" I said.

Shannon cocked her head. With a sly smile and her hand on her hip, she replied, "Anything for me? Really? How about a $500 bonus and some lunch?"

Without missing a beat, I answered, "I *could* write you a check, but it's gonna bounce. But I just stole some donuts from a meeting that I jumped out of early to come here. I just dropped them off in the lounge. I could hook you up with one of those. You get first pick."

Shaking her head, she replied, "You really know how to charm a girl, huh?" while walking toward the lounge. "I'm going for a glazed donut to match my glazed eyes!" she said as she disappeared into the lounge for a moment of sugary happiness.

I pulled back the curtain and was surprised at what I saw. A gentleman of about 80 was smiling back at me. The best way to describe him is that he very much resembled former President Ronald Reagan. Full head of hair, mostly brown, tanned, and pretty fit for his age. He was a handsome guy. "Well, hello there, young man! I hope you're not the undertaker. The rumors of my death are highly exaggerated, although I have at least two ex-wives who would be happy to read that obituary!" This guy was a character.

Playing along, I said, "Now, do I look like an undertaker?"

Without missing a beat, he said, "No, you look more like a lawyer. If you're either, I'm outta here!"

Wow. This man has been sleeping in an ED hallway for two days, and he's smiling and telling jokes. "Actually, I'm one of the nurses here. I'm what they call the clinical manager. I'm here to take you to a better place," I explained.

Chuckling, the man said, "That's what the undertaker says, too!"

Now that was funny. I told him about holding, and explained that it was somewhere between the ED and a bed in a room.

Ever the comedian, he said, "Great, now you sound like a priest. I'm not going to heaven, I'm not going to hell, so more or less, I'm getting sent to purgatory!"

I loved this man. Shaking his hand, I told him my name, and he said, "Pleased to meet you. Call me Sid."

We made the short journey to the holding area, and I helped get him settled. I complimented him on his fitness. He flexed an impressive bicep and said, "You know how I keep these arms so muscular?"

Thinking I was about to get some good fitness advice, I said, "Tell me!"

Sid smiled and said, "I write some big alimony checks! Two a month. I press really hard when I'm writing, and when she tries to take it from my hand, I pull back as hard as I can!"

This guy was a regular Jerry Seinfeld. "No, thanks!" I said. "I'll keep my gym membership!"

He sighed, shrugging his shoulders. "You're smarter than you look! But, to be honest, my exes deserve every penny. I wasn't the best husband."

I was surprised by Sid's sudden seriousness. There was an awkward pause. Noticing my silence, he smiled and said, "Both of my ex-wives became friends with each other. One lives in Dallas and the other in Houston. Isn't that a country song? All my exes live in Texas?" We both laughed.

I started moving Sid's belongings out from under the stretcher. He didn't have much. A bag of clothes and a small, very worn brown leather suitcase. Just then I got paged overhead. I settled Sid in and told him I had to go, but I was sorry to leave him as he was the most fun patient I had met in a long time. His face suddenly got serious. "Would you come back and visit?" Surprised by the sudden change in his tone, I said, "For sure, Sid."

As I walked away, he yelled over my shoulder, "And bring me a bottle of Scotch and a T-bone, medium rare. I ordered that an hour ago. What kind of establishment are you running around here?!?" causing the entire holding department to burst out laughing.

This guy was a hoot.

When my day was over, I called my wife and told her not to wait for me for dinner, that I had some work to catch up on and wanted to help the next shift move out some patients. I also wanted to visit with Sid. I went over to holding and could see him in his bed.

He was staring to his left, looking rather sad. Suddenly he looked up and our eyes met. His whole expression changed. When he saw me, you would've thought I was an old friend he hadn't seen in years.

"Look who it is! My pal Rich," Sid called out with a big grin.

"Well, you look happy to see me!" I said as I sat down.

His expression changed to a pretend scowl. "That was because I thought you had a bottle of Scotch and a T-bone behind your back! What kind of friend shows up empty-handed?"

"I can get you a turkey sandwich and some apple juice," I said apologetically.

"I thought you loved me, Rich!"

We both laughed. "How are you, Sid? Can I get you anything?"

Still smiling, he responded, "Unless you got an extra cancer-free pancreas lying around, I don't need much else."

My smile abruptly left my face. I hadn't really looked at his chart when I moved him to holding in all of the rush, so I didn't know his "clinical status," per se. Ashamed, I said, "Sid, I'm sorry...I..."

"Don't get all mushy on me, kid. It is what it is. We all gotta go sometime." I sat there quietly. I could tell he was not the "pity party" type. Sensing my discomfort, he slapped my arm. "I'm fine. I want to show you something. Now, it's weird I have this with me, but when the ambulance brought me from my house, I was sort of woozy and

I had this next to me, so the paramedics thought I packed a bag for my hospital stay and they grabbed it when they transported me." He pointed at the old leather bag. "Hand that to me."

I grabbed the bag, which was heavier than I recalled. Opening it up, I could see it was full of dozens (if not more) of small leather notebooks. The smell of old leather wafted out of the bag. These were finely made, elegant little notebooks.

"That's my life right there. The secret to my success. My journals. I've been keeping them since before you were born. Probably before your parents were born." Sid handed me one. "Go ahead; open it."

I opened to the first page. The writing was in very neat cursive, the kind of handwriting you don't see anymore. It almost looked like some kind of computer-created font. Perfect. "Wow. Your handwriting is amazing," I said.

"Well, it probably doesn't take much to impress you, since you're used to seeing that doctor handwriting all day long! Read something."

Turning to the first page, I read the date out loud and gasped. "What's wrong?" Sid asked.

"June 20, 1969. That's my birthday!"

Surprised, he said, "Well, what do you know? Talk about a coincidence." He paused. "But then again, I don't believe in those."

Looking up, I replied, "You don't believe in coincidences?"

"Not really," Sid explained. "I think things happen according to some plan. God, I think. I don't think of this world just happening to pop up at exactly the right distance from the sun to allow for life as a 'coincidence.' I've read that the chance of that happening is like a trillion to one or something. I think it was a plan, a divine plan. Something intelligent, some energy, some power. I have my own beliefs about that.

"My successes in life and my failures have all been too amazing and incredible to be just good or bad luck. I think things happen for a reason. You happen to open this exact journal with your exact birthdate? That's pretty nifty. What's it say? What was I writing about as you were gracing us all with your presence?" he asked.

I began to read, "June 20, 1969. I am a grateful man. My son is two years old and spends half his time laughing and the other half giggling. I've never seen a happier little human. I am grateful for doubling my sales this last quarter and for my promotion. The new house is another thing I am grateful for. Three bathrooms! Like the Taj Mahal! Life is good. I make it good. I am grateful today."

I was amazed that Sid had been recording his life since before I was born. It felt like I was holding a piece of history in my hands. I whispered to myself, "This is so cool. These are his journals."

Smirking, Sid responded, "You must've graduated top of your nursing class! Didn't I already tell you that those were my journals?"

Embarrassed at being overheard, I replied, "Second, actually."

"Impressive." He smiled. "I get the second-best nurse in the world taking care of me. I bet the first one would've remembered the Scotch!" Pausing, he said, "Yes, Nurse Einstein, these are my journals. Every day I would write some diary stuff but mostly I would write what I was grateful for."

"Like a gratitude list?" I asked.

Sid looked at me with a deadpan expression. "Are you sure you were second in your class? Was it a really small class?"

"You're a comedian!" I said. "Seriously, is that what these are? You just wrote what you were grateful for?"

"Exactly," he confirmed. "I learned it from an old man I met when I shined shoes.

"You see, I was poor as a kid," he explained. "Not poor like your generation looks at poor. I see 'poor people' all around town with cars and jewelry and cell phones and houses. I am not saying they don't struggle, but in my day, poor was poor. Like, we stole potatoes from old man Bart's stand and ran like hell to the junkyard. We'd make a fire and throw them in and wait until they were roasted, and that would be our breakfast and lunch. I had the same pants for a whole school year. Shoes? My old man would go to car junkyards and strip seats off of old cars to patch our shoes.

"My brother and I shined shoes on the corner, and every penny went to my parents," he added. "I was a smart, energetic kid. Most kids who shined shoes looked like street kids. They couldn't help it. That's all they knew. I figured if I looked clean then maybe I'd attract better customers. I used to go to our kitchen and scrub my face and clean my nails and get my sister to comb my hair. We had a small herb garden off our front stoop, and my mother used to grow mint. I'd grab a handful of mint leaves and chew them up so my breath was clean. Sometimes I even pressed my worn clothes. Anything to get an edge. Oh boy, did I get made fun of by the other shoe shine kids! They used to call me 'Shiny Sidney' and 'Little Lord Sidney.' Luckily I was a scrappy kid and wasn't one to back down."

Sid paused to gather his thoughts, then continued. "Anyway, I got what you might call my big break when I found a more upscale bar about three miles from where we lived. All the other kids crowded around the same joints in our rundown neighborhood. One day I followed a well-dressed man who happened to be passing through our part of town. I think he was lost, but only a few miles away from where he wanted to be—it was like another world.

"Anyway, he went into this bar and I started noticing that all the fellows going in and out looked pretty well heeled. So I dropped my stuff there and within a minute or two had my first customer. Before you know it, I was busy. These guys even tipped me! Then I met him. The man who would change my whole life. He was a gentleman's gentleman. Mr. Colton. What set him apart was that as soon as he sat in my old shoe shine chair, he leaned forward and said, 'What a smart young lad. You picked a good spot. What's your name, child?'

"Understand, in those days, no one cared what a kid's name was. No one ever asked me. They called me 'boy' or 'shoe shine boy.' I told Mr. Colton my name. He put his hand on my shoulder and said, 'Good things will be coming your way, young man. I see a bright future for you.'

"It was like this once a week," Sid continued. "Mr. Colton would find me and take a seat. Every time he would ask me about my grades or what books I was reading. I remember telling him I didn't own any books. He nodded. The next week, he handed me a paper bag after he paid me for my shine. 'Now you have books.' In the bag were *Moby Dick* and the complete works of Thoreau and Emerson. It was a whole new world. I began reading like my life depended on it. Whenever I was shining Mr. Colton's shoes, he would ask me about what I was reading and what I learned. My parents didn't even give me that much interest. They loved me but they were too busy trying to survive.

"Then my whole life changed when Mr. Colton asked me to work in his office. Steady money! He walked me into a clothing store and bought me some pants, shirts, real shoes, and socks. He sent a note home to my parents, complimenting them on raising a 'fine young man' and invited my father to meet him, which he did. Mr. Colton treated my dad with such respect. When I was walking home with my pop after meeting Mr. Colton, Dad told me, 'Kid, that's a gentleman right there. You watch him and learn.'"

Sid took a sip of water, then went on.

"I went to work in Mr. Colton's insurance office: cleaning up, running errands, and doing any odd jobs I could," he recalled. "I was making almost as much as my old man, but more importantly, I was learning. This continued through my school years, and to make a long story short, when I graduated, Mr. Colton put me to work. By that time, I was pretty well versed in everything 'insurance.'

"I learned to sell; I learned about all of the products," Sid reminisced. "I was easily making more than 95 percent of my friends, and probably even their folks. As if this all wasn't enough to change my life, one day Mr. Colton sat me down and showed me one of his journals—kind of like the one you're holding now. He said, 'Sid, life is a lesson, a daily lesson. Lessons can only serve you if they're learned, and one must continue to learn to grow and succeed. I want you to start writing things down every day. Thoughts, dreams, what makes you happy, what stresses you out, and most importantly, what you're grateful for.'

"He shared with me that it is usually a person's natural inclination to recall the things that went wrong, and not so much what went right," Sid added. "He said if you can always maintain a sense of gratitude, you can assure yourself of a successful life. He then handed me a handsomely wrapped package, and within it was my very first journal."

Sid stopped, picked up one of his journals and thumbed through it. For a few moments, he was lost in memory.

"Mr. Colton told me to always be wise with my money but not to scrimp on the journals," he continued. "So at the risk of sounding like a snob, I always bought quality leather ones. From that day forward, I began the life habit of writing down what I am grateful for, even when I am having the worst day."

I was spellbound. Already Sid had told me one of the most fascinating stories I'd heard in a long time. I was so glad I had decided to stay at the hospital and visit with this man after my shift ended. But Sid wasn't finished yet!

Looking up from the journal, Sid said, "Well, to make a long story short, I ended up being the top salesman. As Mr. Colton got older, he handed the whole operation over to me.

"Shortly thereafter, I married my first wife, and life was good. One day Mr. Colton called me to visit him at home. We shared a meal, and then he pulled out some papers for me to look at. He said, 'Sid, this is all going to be yours. I love you like a son. But I warn you, this level of wealth can break a man if he's not careful.'"

Sid smiled a little and shook his head, still amazed by what had transpired so many years ago.

"As I read the paperwork, I realized he was leaving me not only the business, but his estate," he said. "I was stunned. Mr. Colton was a wealthy man. Two years later, as I dried my tears over his coffin, I became a wealthy man too.

"But Mr. Colton was right," Sid added. "The money changed me. Not in great ways. I won't bore you, but I ended up divorced and remarried and then divorced again. My kids keep their distance, and the only time I hear from them is when they want something. But Mr. Colton used to always tell me, 'A life lived perfectly is a perfect impossibility. If you mess up, find a way to make it up. If you feel bad about yourself, find a way to give a gift to another person. For every wrong, do one right, and the odds will always favor you.'"

"So what about the journals?" I asked Sid.

"What about them?" he responded. "I still write in them every day, and every day my list of what I am grateful for grows longer."

Now, I have the worst poker face in the world. So as I, a young man at the time, looked at another, older man with a really bad diagnosis, it was obvious what I was thinking.

Sid smiled. "So what the hell does a guy dying of cancer have to be grateful for, you're asking?"

Embarrassed at being figured out, I stammered, "I'm sorry…but… yeah…I was just thinking…"

He raised his hand to stop me. Looking me up and down, he said, "Well, if I was healthy, I would never have met you. The second-best nurse in his class. What could be better than that?"

Smiling, I responded, "Meeting the first-best?"

Sid let out a surprised laugh and said, "That's a good one, kid! You're learning!"

When I went home that night, Sid was on my mind. What an interesting man. When I came back to work, I was told that he had been moved to a room, which made me happy—at least he was out of holding, or as he had called it, purgatory. That afternoon, when I could finally pull away from the ED, I spoke with the staff caring for him. They told me several serious-looking guys in suits had been coming and going all morning, and that after one visit, Sid seemed really upset.

When I went in to see Sid, he was not his usual happy self. "Hey, kid," he said.

"Hey, Sid, you okay?" I asked. "I heard you had some visitors. Everything alright?"

Looking up, he replied, "Yeah. Lawyers. Mine. My kids'. The exes'. They all want to make sure that they get their share." He sighed and gazed out the window. Then suddenly, his whole energy changed. Turning to me, he smiled and said, "Hey, if it would be okay, I'm gonna call you 'copilot'!"

A little bewildered at the sudden change in subject, I asked, "Why?"

He said, "Because I thought calling you 'number two' might hurt your feelings. But a copilot is also second like you were...so, is that okay?"

I laughed. "Sure, Sid, you can call me whatever you want."

Just then his nurse came in, and I could tell right away she loved Sid. "Speaking of calling, Nurse Fran over here—who is way too young and way too married for me—told me that her mom is recently single and I want to call her...but Fran says her mom needs time to get over her ex. What's that mean? The best way to get over an ex is *me*! Tell her, copilot!"

Fran turned to me. "Copilot?"

Shaking my head, I said, "It's a long story!"

Sid perked up. "No, it's not. Rich was second in his nursing class, so he's like the copilot. I thought 'number two' was too rude. What do you think, Fran?"

Fran let out a loud laugh. "Number two? Now that would be fun!"

"Don't even think about it, Fran!" I warned.

"Pinkie swear!" she said. "Your secret is safe with me!" She smiled as she left the room with a twirl that was more dramatic than necessary.

Sid and I talked for awhile, and I could tell he didn't want to discuss lawyers or cancer. Who could blame him? (I have some great lawyer friends, and they'd agree!)

A week or so went by, and my visits with Sid were the highlight of my day. I could tell he was having an impact on others as well—it was just a natural side effect of his positive energy. He asked me to talk to his doctors and help him with a few issues. I learned that Sid was much sicker than he appeared. He was in the true end stages of cancer, and although he was admitted to a regular floor, the care team was changed to more of a hospice palliative care model. Sid started to have more and more pain every day. On some visits he slept, and I held his hand or just sat with him while doing paperwork.

I knew of him having only a few visitors. They were mostly lawyers with more paperwork, but there also was a mechanic who worked on Sid's cars, his housekeeper, and some golf buddies. Every one of them shared with me what a great guy Sid was and how sad he was that his kids were so distant. One day, when Sid was awake and lucid, he handed me a phone number. "It's my son. Can you call him? I want to talk to him."

I dialed the number and a woman answered in a formal-sounding voice. I asked for Sid's son by name and told her who I was and why

I was calling. It was apparent she was an employee of the son by her responses. "One moment," she said, and I was put on hold. "He said he will call later. Thank you."

He never did.

Around Christmas, I was scheduled for vacation. Before I left, I visited Sid to say goodbye and told him that I'd see him when I got back. He looked up at me and with an uncharacteristically serious tone said, "No, you won't, copilot. I'm checking out of here soon." I knew what he meant, and I also learned long ago that when a patient says something like that, they're usually right.

My eyes started to tear up. Sid grabbed my hand, and looking right at me he said, "Don't cry, copilot...I'll pay my bill." Typical Sid. But this broke up the sadness.

He reached over to his bedside table and handed me a package wrapped in tissue. "Open it, copilot. Merry Christmas." I did. It was a really nice leather journal. Apparently he had sent one of his friends to purchase it for him while he was in the hospital.

"Sid...I...don't know what to say."

"How about you just say thanks and promise you'll make a habit of writing down what you are grateful for every day, and then pass the lesson on to someone else. The more the merrier. Just do that. Please promise—that's the most important thing. That you pass this on," he said with an unusually serious tone I had never heard from him before.

"You got it, Sid, I will. Thanks. It's beautiful."

He looked at me for a second. "Well?" he asked.

"Well what?" I asked, still surprised by the cool gift.

"Geez. I'm surprised you weren't 20th in your class...What's in the bag you got next to you with the red ribbon and the tag that says, 'Sid'? I may be old and dying, but I am not blind and stupid!"

Laughing, I handed him the Christmas bag. "It had better be that bottle of Scotch," he commented as he tore out the tissue like a little kid on Christmas morning. Then his smile disappeared. At first I thought I had upset him. I had never seen him looking sad, except for the two brief moments when his son didn't take his call and when he mentioned the lawyers' visit. Then Sid closed his eyes, and I could tell he was fighting back tears.

"Copilot. Thanks. You're first in my class. Give me a hug." I hugged Sid, and then he pulled back and proudly placed his copies of *Moby Dick* and the complete works of Emerson and Thoreau on his bedside table.

"I figured you might like to catch up on some reading," I said.

He smiled. "That I would."

We spent a little more time talking, and then Sid started having some pain again. His nurse brought him some meds, and he of course had to show off his books and wouldn't let her leave until he told her the entire story of me being second in my class.

We hugged, and as I walked out, he called me back. "Hey, copilot!"

Turning, I said, "Yes, Sid?"

"Be grateful every day, kid. Promise you'll pass it on. What did that nurse say the other day when she made you a promise?"

Remembering what Fran had said to me, I laughed and responded, "Pinkie promise!"

Sid waved me over and he stuck up his pinkie. "Pinkie promise?"

Connecting my pinkie to Sid's, I replied, "Pinkie promise."

I took one last look at Sid as he dozed off. I felt grateful for knowing him.

On Christmas morning I called my ED to wish them a Merry Christmas and to thank them for working. I tried not to rub it in that this year was my Christmas off, and I mentioned that I wanted to be connected to Sid's room to say Merry Christmas. One of my staff told me that the morning supervisor, a good friend of mine who was just coming on, had asked to speak to me.

When my friend got to the phone, she informed me that Sid had passed away just after midnight on Christmas Eve. I wasn't on his chart as "family," and the staff working that night didn't know about my friendship with him—so no one had called me. She felt bad, but I understood.

My friend went on to say that a lawyer had come (yes, they work on Christmas too, apparently!) and showed her paperwork giving him the legal right to take Sid's body and all of his possessions. She said that there was a suitcase containing some leather books as well as a few novels, the ones I had given to Sid. The lawyer apparently didn't want these and told her she could dispose of them. She knew of my friendship with Sid and asked if I wanted her to put them aside for me. I thanked her and asked her to please place them in my office.

"Do you know if there were any plans for a service or anything? Did he leave a card?" I asked. My friend read me Sid's lawyer's card info. I thanked her and hung up. I can't explain why, because I am an emotional guy, but I don't recall crying. I felt sad, for sure. But there was a part of me that knew Sid was truly at peace.

Later that day, I called Sid's lawyer and left a message inquiring about his service. To my surprise, a woman called me back a few hours later and informed me that there would be no service. Sid was to be cremated as per his family's request, and his ashes were to be spread at sea later that week. She thanked me for my concern and wished me well.

Before she hung up, I asked, "Will anyone be there for the spreading of the ashes?"

She paused, probably surprised by the audacity of the question. "No. That wasn't the wish of the family. Thanks. Have a happy holiday." And she hung up.

When I returned to work a few days later, I made sure to arrive at my office very early. There was the box. My office smelled like fine leather from all of those journals. I began reading a few. Sure enough, day after day, through good and bad times, this man had written about what he was grateful for. Looking through the box, I came across Sid's final journal and turned to the last page. The date was 12/23. He listed the names of physicians and nurses he was grateful for. And then the last line read:

"I am grateful that I have learned to be grateful no matter what. As the end nears, I hope I kept my promise to you, Mr. Colton. I passed it along like you said. I am feeling angry and hurt that my kids have left me as they have, but I forgive them and I love them and I hope they do good things…no, great things with the money I am leaving them. I am grateful for my friend Rich, and I know he will keep the promise, the pinkie promise of all things! Today I am grateful for my life. I am grateful for a peaceful death. I will not be sad or angry for anything. I will instead be grateful."

I closed the journal and stared out of my office window. I was amazed at these words and that I was a part of Sid's story, his incredible story. Then the phone rang and it was back to work.

Around 5:30 p.m. as I was packing up, our triage nurse called and told me that there was a man demanding to see me out front. She said he was a lawyer. "Send him back." A well-dressed man in his 50s, who looked as if he walked straight off a movie set where he had been playing the role of Perfect Palm Beach Lawyer, handed me a card.

"Mr. Bluni, my colleague was here on Christmas morning, and there seems to have been an error. I was told there was a box of the deceased's records that were incorrectly left behind and that somehow you are in possession of them."

I said, "Well, not really records per se, but Sid's personal journals. Yes, they're right here." Looking over at the box, the lawyer handed me a document authorizing him to take "any and all of the deceased's personal belonging or effects."

He explained, "You see, there is a dispute among the family about the estate, and we are hoping that Sid left further instructions in these books."

I knew the lawyer was more right than he realized about the "instructions," but they weren't going to be what he or the family was hoping for. Reluctantly I handed the box over. The lawyer seemed relieved that I put up no fight. As he left, I stopped him and said, "Would you please make sure his kids read the last page of the last journal, and if they won't, would you at least please tell them that Sid loved them?"

The lawyer looked stunned, as he was obviously not paid $400 an hour to deliver love messages. However, after a moment, his face softened and he said, "I will do that. Thanks." As he whipped out of my office with the open box in hand, I got one more whiff of old leather and felt as if Sid was patting me on the head. I could almost hear his voice saying, "Thanks, copilot!"

After the lawyer was gone, I felt my anger begin to rise. At least I think that's what it was. I was mad that Sid's kids couldn't care less about their father, and that they probably wouldn't read these journals. Instead, they would just be used to fight over money.

Then I remembered what Sid had taught me. I opened up my own journal and began to write down all of the things I was grateful for that day, including the fact that I met a man who changed my life and handed me not only a gift, but a duty to pass on that gift.

And, hopefully, I just did. After all it was a pinkie promise!

Gratitude is more than a cutesy thing that New Agers and mega-church pastors use to sound "spiritual." It's the real deal. I personally believe that gratitude is the most important thing we can "do" to effect change in our lives. There are many ways to "use" gratitude, and I have written about them in blog posts, Facebook posts, and in previous books. I talk about gratitude in the literally thousands of presentations I have done over the last several years. I always will.

Gratitude should not be complicated. Like the steak I hope to someday share with Sid when I meet him again, it should be prepared simply and enjoyed thoroughly. Here are some tips to help you (and your team) start your own gratitude habit:

1. Find a way, any way, to include gratitude in every day. A journal is a great way to do this—so go on, get a notebook! It doesn't have to be fancy like Sid's; it can be as simple as a spiral-bound notebook. If you want to save some trees, go virtual and keep the list on your iPhone or other piece of technology. Just challenge yourself to record at least one thing (or three, or five) that you are thankful for each day. I have heard many times that a life worth living is a life worthy of being written down. Keeping a gratitude journal is a wonderful way to honor your life and point it in the right direction.

Don't worry if you find yourself repeating the same items from time to time. Reflecting on why you're consistently thankful for a particular coworker, for example, will improve your working relationship!

And bonus: When you're having a bad day or feel like you're losing your way—when you want to pack up your "princess suitcase" and walk away from a difficult situation—looking back through your gratitude journal is a fantastic way to boost your mood and reconnect to your inspiration.

2. Create a gratitude chalkboard at work. At the end of each shift, ask the off-going team to write one word or a short sentence describing something they are grateful for so that the oncoming shift can read it. Then rinse and repeat! It creates a very positive focus and is also an excellent way to publicly reward team members whose commitment, attitude, or actions deserve recognition.

3. Tell others about your gratitude. Try this: Whenever someone asks you, "How are you doing?" don't respond with "fine" or "okay." Reply, "I am grateful!" When I do this, 98 percent of the time I get a great response. (The other 2 percent of the time I get weird looks or rolled eyes...but hey, why be normal?) Usually, people smile and some even ask me, "Really? Why?" and I tell them. Sometimes they share right back. I have had flight attendants, hotel workers, taxi drivers, valets, food servers, and toll booth attendants tell me that I "made their day." Some even shared, "I'm going to start answering like that!" With all of the negativity and craziness of this world, why not share a little gratitude? It's the gift that keeps on giving.

See? Simple. Gratitude is a journey. It takes you to amazing places within your spirit. You are the pilot steering that plane. (Or in my case, the copilot!)

CHAPTER

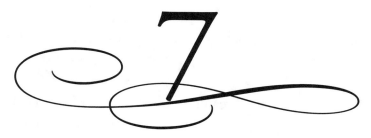

7

WHY ISN'T SHE DEAD YET?

End-of-life issues bring out the best and worst in people. (Nurses know this better than anyone!) That's why, as the director of risk management, I frequently assisted my team, patients, and family members with end-of-life issues. These issues were rarely cut and dry, always emotional, and often challenging.

I remember one patient in particular: an 80-year-old woman named Mrs. Cohen. After being in the ICU for a few days, her condition worsened and she was now completely dependent upon a ventilator. She also had a husband who was usually accompanied by a paid caregiver. The caregiver was—how should I say this?—overly involved in many ways. And Mr. Cohen himself was an angry person. There's no other way to describe him.

Mr. Cohen and his wife had been patients many times in the past, and while she was a kind and gracious woman, he and his caregiver were screamers. While working in my office (which was 30 yards away down a hallway and behind two thick doors), I could often hear them screaming from the lobby when they were having one of their fits.

Lots of things set Mr. Cohen and his hired caregiver, Bev, off. The room was too cold. Screaming. The room was too warm. Screaming. The cafeteria was opened too late. Screaming. The food was "too ethnic" (yes, they actually said that). Screaming. The staff were "too ethnic" (yes, that too!). Screaming. I hated when they screamed at the staff, and I am not one to allow *anyone* to abuse my staff.

I won't bore you with too many details, but trust me when I say we did everything we could to correct Mr. Cohen and Bev's behavior, including involving security, requiring "behavioral contracts" (yeah, that was a winner), and even once accusing Bev of trespassing. Each time, she and Mr. Cohen would beg and plead and promise to "be nice." Even though they were a nightmare to deal with, they never crossed the line to "violent or dangerous," so they were always allowed to return—usually because Mrs. Cohen was brought by fire rescue, and even if we wanted to we couldn't turn her or them away.

Eventually I made it my "job" to deal with these two, which I know my friends and staff appreciated. Mr. Cohen and Bev were told that under no circumstances were they to raise their voices or disrespect the staff. They agreed that if they had an issue, they would come see me. If I wasn't in my office, I would be called. It was the least I could do. It wasn't fun, but it was always interesting.

On this particular admission, it was obvious that Mrs. Cohen was in the end stages. She was a sweet lady, and the staff lovingly cared for her. For the most part, Mr. Cohen and Bev were respectful. I was told by the staff that Mr. Cohen was mostly not happy with the fact that his wife was in the hospital at all, because in his words, "It was a pain in the butt [not the exact word he used] to have to visit every day," and that "if I wanted to visit a vegetable, I'd grow cabbage in my backyard."

What a prince, huh? I can only imagine what life was like for that poor woman. She and Mr. Cohen had kids from out of town who, because of financial issues, couldn't travel to see their mom. However, they called every day, and many times her caregiver or I was there to put the phone to her ear so they could tell her they loved her. The Cohens' son told me that Mr. Cohen was always pretty mean but that he never bullied Mrs. Cohen; she always kept him in line. I was relieved to hear that.

One day the physician taking care of Mrs. Cohen visited me and told me that she had worsened significantly. Apparently Mr. Cohen, as her healthcare surrogate and with her living will in hand (or as the doctor described, "waving it in my face"), wanted to shut off the vent and let her pass peacefully.

Along with Mrs. Cohen's team of caregivers, I waited on Mr. Cohen to arrive and went over, in detail, what we could and couldn't do. We also made sure we answered his questions. Bev was there; she frequently interrupted and made inappropriate comments, as was her norm. Mr. Cohen ended the meeting by saying, "You people talk too damn much and I'm hungry. Just shut off the vent and be done with this. I got things to do. What do I need to sign?" That was that, I guess.

I asked him if he wanted to say goodbye before we removed the vent. He looked at me like I was crazy. "I'm so glad I won't have to talk to you anymore, Mr. Bluni."

Can you feel the love? He then told Bev to take him to lunch.

We were sort of thrown off by Mr. Cohen's behavior, but it wasn't that surprising. I called the Cohen kids and had each of them tell Mrs. Cohen they loved her as I held the phone to her ear. I could hear them sobbing through the receiver, and it broke my heart.

We did all the usual things you do when you remove a vent. And much to our surprise, Mrs. Cohen kept breathing. Like, for a long time. I'm leaving a lot of clinical information out, but suffice it to say, Mrs. Cohen was not ready to leave. She was actually pretty stable and breathing well on her own. What a tough lady! I guess you couldn't be a shrinking violet while married to her husband.

After a period of time, we tried calling Mr. Cohen. No answer. We tried calling Bev. No answer. This went on for a few hours. Finally we got through to Bev. I told her that, basically, Mrs. Cohen surprised us all and was breathing rather comfortably on minimal oxygen and was even waking up a little bit.

Multiple choice question time! Did Bev:
    A. Cry with joy?
    B. Ask me to explain Mrs. Cohen's hemodynamic status?
    C. Scream?

Yep. Screamed. I was told that she and Mr. Cohen would be there as soon as he finished lunch. (How long does lunch take?)

They showed up a little while later and went straight to the floor. Mr. Cohen screamed at everyone he could: physicians, nurses, pharmacy techs, EVS workers, and even passing visitors. Awesome. I wanted to take the drama off the staff's plate and away from the ICU, so I asked him and Bev to be brought to my office.

I greeted the disruptive duo in the lobby and began to walk them toward my office, but when I invited them in, Mr. Cohen refused. He began to scream at me in my office corridor with my staff and a few of my suitemates in attendance for the whole opera.

"What kind of dump are you running here, Bluni? I took my wife off of life support. She was supposed to be dead, she's not, and I have to come back here, interrupting my lunch, and find you bunch of Neanderthals brushing her hair and acting like everything is peachy? What the hell is going on here?"

I calmly interrupted him and tried my best to explain the situation. I told Mr. Cohen that while the clinical team felt strongly that his wife was at an end stage, she was obviously stronger than we thought and she had surprised us all with her tenacity. It even looked like she would continue to improve. All of her medical team was calling it a miracle. Yeah, let's just say my attempt at being Dr. Phil wasn't working.

Mr. Cohen screamed even more, punctuated with a lot of "uh-huhs" and "you tell hims" from Bev. Then he capped off his rant with this gem: "You idiots can't do anything right. You can't even make someone die. You'd think you could at least do that. What's so hard about that?"

I said, "Mr. Cohen, we are not in the habit of euthanizing people. That's not what we do. Your wife surprised us all. No one thought she'd be able to breathe on her own. We told you all that we knew, and this was not something we could foresee. What would you like me to do to make this better for you? How can I help?"

I swear he looked at me and gave me a grin that reminded me of the Grinch Who Stole Christmas—*before* his heart grew three sizes.

"Apologize that my wife is still alive!"

You could hear the collective gasp from my colleagues standing nearby. But I'm a nurse. It takes a lot to shock me. "You want me to apologize to you because your wife is not dead?" I asked flatly.

Bev responded, "That's what the man said." I didn't grace her with even so much as a glance. I locked gazes with Mr. Cohen, and the witnesses all agreed that he must've seen something different in my eyes. They all said he actually looked somewhere between nervous and embarrassed, which was definitely a first for him.

I repeated myself: "You want me to apologize because we failed to end your wife's life? Is that what you need right now, sir?"

He muttered, "Yes."

"Mr. Cohen, I have never done this before and I'm sure I will never do it again, but on behalf of myself and this hospital, I apologize to you that your wife did not pass away. Is that what you wanted to hear, sir?"

"Yes," he said. Bev opened her mouth. I didn't even look at her, but held up one finger. Heaven only knows what kind of inappropriate comment I was putting off, but she closed her mouth. It snapped shut like a crocodile.

"May I add one other thought, sir?" I asked.

"Yes," Mr. Cohen answered reluctantly.

"We are caregivers. We care. We care about your wife and we care about you. We don't put human beings down like racehorses with broken legs, sir. We are not in the business of ending lives but saving them. When we can't save a life, we do all we can to make sure that person's transition is as loving, caring, and respectful as possible. We work every day, 24-7, at that. Some we win, and some we lose. But we always care.

"So while I offered you the apology you wanted, I won't apologize for the hard work and loving care this team has provided. You won't get that from me. Now that you have what you wanted, I need to get on with the business of healthcare. If you'd like to go back up and see your wife, we will be happy to arrange that, and you may spend as much or as little time with her as you want, but sir, you will speak to and treat each person with the respect they deserve. I want you to be crystal clear about that. If you have an issue, a gripe, or a problem, you come see me. Are we clear, sir?"

I wish I could tell you that Mr. Cohen had some great epiphany and fell to his knees with a new perspective—like Ebenezer Scrooge after being visited by his ghosts and seeing the error of his ways—but no.

He just responded, "Crystal clear. Bev, take me home." And they left. Just like that.

Mrs. Cohen improved over the next few days. She even woke up, ate a little, and was able to talk to her kids on the phone. We called her "Our Miracle," and she loved that. She asked the staff to tell her husband that she didn't want him to visit. She allowed Bev to visit once or twice, but soon announced that she was too tired and asked Bev to leave. After Bev had departed, Mrs. Cohen said, "I wasn't too tired. I just didn't want to see her."

Mrs. Cohen bought plane tickets for her kids. They visited and stayed with their dad. I met them and we hugged. They were so grateful and so sweet. They told me that their dad couldn't care less and didn't even ask for Mrs. Cohen. They shared with me that he was always a distant and unkind man and had gotten worse over the years. They kept him updated, but he just nodded and went back to watching TV.

The oldest son also shared with me that he fired Bev. He found out she had taken a few hundred dollars by using Mr. Cohen's ATM card without permission. The police were called, and the son was pretty sure that Bev would be arrested. Wonder if she screamed at the cops? The Cohen children hired a new home aide whom they liked much better (although honestly, Bev set the bar pretty low!).

I am glad that Mrs. Cohen had that time with her kids. Despite her miraculous improvement, she was still a very sick woman and no one was under the illusion that she was going home. Four days after her kids left, Mrs. Cohen died in her sleep. Unlike what I assume her life was like with Mr. Cohen, it was very peaceful.

For years after this whole episode, my coworkers teased me about the fact that I was so good at apologizing that I probably *am* the only healthcare worker in the world who has apologized for saving someone's life. But this type of stuff is reality.

I write books about inspiration and spend a lot of my life speaking all over North America—not because I think our lives as nurses are roses, chocolate, and rainbows, but because I *know* it's often the opposite. Yes, nursing is the most amazing and inspiring profession out there, but it is also tough. Look, I'm real and I have been in this healthcare world for many years. It's okay to say that.

Here's the truth: We deal with really outrageously difficult people sometimes. I didn't say "all of the time" or even "most of the time," because we know that's not true. Honestly, for every 50 to 100 patients you have, only one or two are truly, legitimately mean and difficult, right? And let's be honest, we deal with people when they are sick and at their worst. Even a normally "nice" person may not be at their best when we encounter them! Sometimes, though, it feels like somebody opened up the cages at the "mean zoo" and let all of the angry monkeys out.

People can be tough to deal with. I've been there, my fellow nurse. I have had people punch me, pull guns on me, call me the worst names, wish disease and death upon me, and threaten my loved ones. I have worked in some tough places and dealt with some tough things. I promise you that I am far from perfect, but most of the time I rose above these incidents and people and walked away, sometimes with my heart pounding and my palms sweaty, but always with my head held high. Because for every one of the Mr. Cohens I have crossed paths with, there were 500 Mrs. Cohens.

I am saying this only because I want you to know I get it. My organization, Studer Group®, gets it too. We just choose not to exclusively focus on what's wrong and what's negative, because that would be too easy. Sure, we *could* look at that "truly difficult" 1-2 percent, throw up our hands, and adopt the whole "people stink" attitude. Soon, we'd see "difficult" in every request and "mean" in every complaint. It would become second nature to blame others and hold no personal accountability. (We've all known coworkers like this.) Personally, I think this attitude is a total cop out. Moreover, it's certainly not the behavior we want to see in our staff or the type of care we want to give to our patients.

So, once we acknowledge the truth that there are unstable and mean people out there, then what? How do we not let them drain our inspiration? How *do* we stay motivated and positive when we encounter people like Mr. Cohen, with whom you can do nothing right... ever? As I've said, it's no fun and usually quite uninspiring to care for people like him. (But as Sinatra said, "That's life!") Here are a few strategies:

1. Remind yourself that each patient (and each visitor!) is fighting a difficult battle. I have heard it said many times and in many different ways that you should always be kind to people, because you never know what battle they are fighting. This may sound weird, but as nurses we have an advantage here. Think about a "Mr. Cohen" you are caring for. You DO know, to a great extent, what that patient's battle is. It's no mystery. Their battle is cancer, or a fracture impeding their mobility, or being out of work because of their hospitalization. It's right there on their chart. They are fighting a battle right before your eyes, and you are in the trenches with them.

When you are in a battle with someone, fighting alongside them, it is sometimes easy to get caught in the crossfire. In battles there can be incidences called "friendly fire" when an ally accidentally attacks or fires on another ally. It is unintended, but it happens. Soldiers say that friendly fire can be caused by what's called "the fog of war." Simply put, "the fog of war" is the confusion and intensity and urgency and quick changes that make war what it is.

We are fighting on the frontlines with our patients. Often we are alongside them for the most difficult battles of their lives. They are experiencing strong emotions, fears, and drama that create a sort of "healthcare fog of war." Therefore, we are sometimes recipients of friendly fire, if you will. Have you ever had a patient or family member "go off" on you, and then return or call you the next day to apologize? I think we all have.

Understand, to paraphrase what many of us have heard in our dating days, "It's not you; it's them!" Maybe more specifically, it's the cancer or pain or fear or anxiety that is contributing to the behavior you are experiencing. So, take a breath. Sometimes the best thing to do is acknowledge it in the moment. "I know you're scared. I get it. I am on your side. Let me help you." (To be real, that tactic may work only 5 to 10 percent of the time, but that's at least better than 0 percent!)

So, let's recap:
- Step one: Tell yourself that this isn't personal; the patient's battle is what's probably causing their difficult behavior.
- Step two: Be honest, calm, and sincere, and acknowledge to the patient that you understand that they're facing a battle. Sometimes what people—even ones who may seem "diffi-cult"—want to hear is, "I get it, I feel for you, I see what you

are dealing with, I am here for you…" Hopefully this alone makes an impact.

2. Help others tap into hope. Sometimes what people are really looking for when they're acting out is hope. So in addition to acknowledging that you see what a patient is going through, if possible, give them hope.

You might say, "I know it seems like it's never going to get better. But I have seen literally hundreds of people dealing with what you are right now, and I can promise you from my 20 years of nursing experience that you will see the nausea subside within a few hours. We will get you better. Hang in there with me." At Studer Group we call this "Key Words at Key Times." It's really not rocket science, and it's really not a "fake scripted" thing. Not at all.

When people are given a light at the end of the tunnel or a sign that "this too shall pass," then you are reducing their anxiety. This opens the door for them to feel a sense of peace. We can't be anxious and peaceful at the same time. It's not possible.

When I am anxious, I cannot think clearly and I am raw. I always say that it is a short trip from anxious to angry. Let me say that again: It is a short trip from anxious to angry. Make sense? Often, when people are anxious, it doesn't take much to set them off. If we can reduce a patient's anxiety, we make it less likely that they'll become angry and therefore act out.

But there's one important caveat: Give hope only when there *is* hope. When I was a student, I read an old EMT training manual that included a chapter about discussing bad news with a patient's loved ones in the event of a death or serious injury. One sentence in particular made my friends and me burst out laughing: "In the case of a total decapitation, do not give the family false hope." I mean, really? But you get the point. When I refer to hope, I am referring to any *realistic* "ray of light" you can give when someone is scared.

In most cases there *is* something you can say to make a patient less anxious. When a human being is suffering, hurting, or scared they want to know that there will be a "break" and "end." Sometimes this knowledge will turn things around.

3. Tag team when you can. Let's be honest: There are people who will think you are an angel, and there are people who will think you have horns and a pitchfork. That's normal and to be expected. Sometimes people just clash. Maybe you remind that patient of her ex-husband's new wife. Maybe you wore a cologne that reminded another patient of their former business partner who stole all the money and took off for Argentina. If you think an issue like that is at play, perhaps there is an opportunity to switch patients with a colleague.

I have been on both sides of this solution. For instance, my buddy was clashing with a patient, so I took over and all was good. The next day a family member took a strong dislike to me (Shocking, right? Not really…), so I switched with someone and all was good.

Once again, there's a caveat: Don't abuse the switch-up strategy. It's not fair to just call a tag team for any and every "tough" case. But used wisely, it *is* a realistic and honest option. Sometimes it's *not* them…it's you!

4. Have a plan to help you deal with true "Mr. Cohens." I'll be honest: Sometimes there's nothing you can do to influence the behavior of a difficult patient or loved one. None of the previous tactics I've shared worked with Mr. Cohen and his evil henchwoman, Bev. My team and I tried Key Words at Key Times. We switched caregivers. We tried kindness, empathy, therapeutic communication, boundary setting, chocolate, humor, begging, pleading, and Jedi mind tricks. Nothing. Worked.

But listen to me, please: This is not the norm. This is the exception. At one time or another ALL of us have had a patient or family described to us as being "impossible to please" or have been told that "nothing works…we have tried everything." And then after 30 minutes with you they're writing letters to the mayor about how awesome you are and bringing you coffee every morning. So, for *most* people, there is *something* that works. Right now, I'm *not* talking about those people.

We live in the real world. There are people out there who were mad when the doctor or midwife slapped them on the butt and will stay mad until they are lowered into the ground and have that first handful of dirt thrown on their casket 95 years later. They were mad on all of the days in between, at almost every person they encountered. Do you think Mr. Cohen was mean only to me and the staff but was a sweetheart to his server in a restaurant, the person repairing his refrigerator at home, or a neighbor walking by? Of course not. Even his own family, including his dying wife, shared that he was a deeply unhappy and difficult person, and had always been that way! As a wise guru once said, "Haters gonna hate." It is what it is.

So then what? How *do* you deal with true "Mr. Cohens"—those who are truly impossible or hateful? Here's my advice:

- **Strive to stay professional.** You can never be unprofessional or disrespectful—and why should you be? Then the other person wins, right? Once you step out of line, they get to do what most truly despicable people do: play the victim card. And you will always lose. You know this to be true. Remember, you don't have control over many things in life. Not the weather, not what another person says or does, and not who rolls through the doors at work. But what you *do* have complete control over is how you choose to think about those things and therefore how you react. If I am mean, angry, loud, and abusive, why should you be the same? Is that who you want to be? I mean for real. No. No. No!

- **Walk away when necessary.** Pull yourself away from that negative energy. Sometimes you'll have to do this literally. We've all been in situations where we had to walk away to cool off so that we wouldn't say or do something we'd regret. It's also important that you set boundaries, because you never deserve to be abused. And if the situation is in any way threatening or violent, then you need to put your safety first and foremost.

- **Don't beat yourself up for not being able to improve the situation.** As I've said, there are people who not only can't be pleased but on some deep level don't want to be. Their whole persona is built around being mean. You are not going to fix them. And it's not your fault. So don't carry that burden!

- **As Shakespeare wrote, "To thine own self be true."** Be the inspired, kind, mature, professional that you are. Don't pivot, don't deviate, don't lower yourself to the pettiness that is being thrown at you. Do what you can do. Do your job and do it well. Don't get thrown off your game. A professional athlete will tell you that they play better when they are facing a tougher opponent. So, put your game face on. Be the leader. Be the energy you want around you. Give yourself some peace.

- **Don't give difficult people an all-access pass to your mood.** On your break, don't continue to focus on this person or issue. Don't take them home with you in your conversations. Don't vent about them to your peers. The more energy you give them, the more powerful they become.

  Instead, go meditate or listen to your favorite tunes. Eat something that makes you happy. Sit next to the funniest nurse you know at lunch and get an endorphin rush from some laughter. Understand that you are dealing with a person who is probably in some deep psychological pain, so love them and care for them to the best of your ability. If you follow any type of spiritual path, pray for them or send them good vibes…and then let them go.

- **Give yourself hope!** This won't last forever. That difficult patient or family member will leave someday. Your shift will end at some point.

- **Ask for support when you need it.** Trust me, if a patient or loved one is truly as bad as all that, a lot of others will know. Get the support of your leader and your team. Work together. An old proverb once said: A bundle of sticks is harder to break than a single twig. If there was one thing that *did* work in the case of Mr. Cohen, it was that the nurses on the floor, their managers, me, and many others supported one other.

  People and times can be tough, but I believe that nurses and other healthcare workers are tougher. I will always believe that, because I have seen it over and over in my sisters and brothers who inspire me every day with their tenacity, spirit, and power. And I have seen it in me! Sometimes, like you, I just need to be reminded.

- **Look for hidden gifts.** When I think of all of the stress and pain Mr. Cohen put me and the team through, I also realize that there were gifts hidden in all that upheaval. I was able to participate in helping Mrs. Cohen say goodbye to her kids and grandkids. She and I laughed together more than a few times, and I marveled at her ability to be a light despite the darkness of her spouse. I also got to see that even when faced with an impossible-to-please person, I could, for the most part, keep my cool and do what was right. Remembering that truth about myself has since helped me navigate other difficult situations.

- **Consciously choose to stay inspired.** You and I know that sometimes life can be unfair, disorganized, stressful, and not nice. But hopefully that is not how it always is for you. Hopefully you are reading this book because you are the type of person who chooses to see the possibility of inspiration in what you do and who you are, in spite of the fact that there are people, moments, and even periods of time that seem to be anything but inspiring. But even those—maybe especially those—give us our greatest opportunities to be better.

You see, being inspired doesn't mean you've lived a perfect life where everyone was always nice, you always got exactly what you wanted for your birthday, the busses were all on time, and every lotto ticket you bought was a winner. Being inspired is a *choice*. It is a state of mind YOU and you alone decide to adopt, regardless of the actions or words of others…because those words and actions are theirs, not yours! So let the anger and unhappiness be theirs, not yours.

Let me say that again: Your inspiration is not dependent upon the whims and moods of another person. It will always be your birthright as a nurse. Never surrender it to anyone. And never apologize because you wouldn't let your inspiration die!

CHAPTER

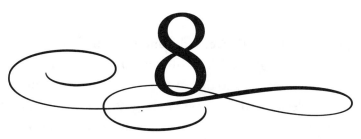

8

YOU GOT THIS...YOU'RE BATMAN

We always remember firsts. First kiss, first job, first best friend. My first best friend was David. We met when I was around 12 years old and David was 14, and we were inseparable for years. We were total nerds together. We both were obsessed with movies, science fiction, Dungeons & Dragons, and comic books.

We *loved* our comics! Our favorite superhero, we both agreed, was Batman. We reasoned, in the way that only the wisest 12- and 14-year-olds could, that he was superior to most other superheroes. He wasn't an alien. He didn't need a magical ring or to be bitten by a radioactive spider, and he had no special mutant powers. He was a regular guy who worked hard and used what he had to become totally awesome. We loved Batman, and he was a big part of our lives. Some of our friends even referred to us as "The Dynamic Duo"! Whenever one of us would be bummed or have a bad day, the other would always say some version of, "You got this...you're Batman!" as encouragement.

David and I were both "theater kids" and were in tons of shows together. He was so talented and truly the funniest person I have ever met. As teenagers we used to dream together about what our futures would be. We decided that we were both going to be ridiculously famous. David would be a legendary stage actor and would win a Tony or two. Sometimes he would practice his speech where he would thank me, because I was going to be the next Al Pacino. I would win an Oscar the same year he won a Tony and I would thank him in *my* speech, too. He would drive a black Ferrari while I'd have a white one.

The only thing bigger than our dreams was our love for each other as brothers. I spent the most formative years of my life with David. He was fearless and loyal to a fault. If you talked about me, it had better be for a good reason, because he would defend me to the death. He was truly the best friend a guy could have. Even today in my 40s, I still can see the influence this friendship had on my life.

Eventually I was accepted into a theater program at NYU and left Miami. David started hanging out with a different group of friends, and we drifted apart. If you're from a younger generation, allow me to point out that keeping in touch 30 years ago was a little different. With today's social media, email, cell phones, and tech, it's so easy. Back then you had a phone number and an address, and hopefully a mutual acquaintance connected to that person. If someone moved, even once, or that connection left town, it was easy to lose touch.

Over the years I would occasionally visit Miami and always tried to find David. Sometimes I could. Sometimes I couldn't. I learned later on from several third-party sources that he had fallen on some challenging times (which made it clear, in hindsight, why I was unable to locate him). David had lost both of his parents, two beautiful human beings I loved as second parents when I was a kid, and his life had taken some dark turns.

Connecting with David became even harder over the years. Once in a while I would get lucky and locate an address or phone number, and when we talked, it was like we were still two kids hanging out in each other's rooms. Whenever we hung out, David liked to focus on those times, and I could tell he was uncomfortable talking about his life in more recent days. That was fine. We would just recall stories and laugh. His memory was uncanny. I didn't even argue with him when we disagreed, because he remembered everything perfectly. He was like a living scrapbook. And he still had every picture and poster from every show we ever performed. I showed him that, while I had lost dozens of photo albums over the years, I always kept two pictures: one photo of him and me dressed up for Halloween when we were around 13 and 15, and a sketch he drew (he was an amazing artist!) of my teenage favorite pop star, Adam Ant! (Don't laugh; it was the '80s!)

When I moved back to Miami from NYC in my later 20s, I was able to find David less and less. The years passed like leaves blowing on an October evening. David, my first best friend, had all but disappeared. While I thought of him frequently, I only infrequently ran into people who knew him. They all said the same thing: "I haven't seen him in years." And for awhile, neither did I. Marriage, my father's passing, nursing school, children, and jobs all filled in the gaps once occupied by a "best friend."

More years went by. And then in April 2015, while I was boarding a plane, David just popped into my head. It occurred to me, *Facebook!*

Maybe he's on Facebook! David has a very common name, so finding him took a little bit of time, but then I saw his picture! It was him! I immediately messaged my old friend, and to my joy and surprise he responded in seconds. He wrote that he missed his best friend and asked if I could call him right away. I promised to do so as soon as my plane landed.

Within a few hours the phone was ringing, and I was about to talk to my long-lost brother. I was psyched. After a few seconds of small talk, I asked, "How are you, buddy?"

Without hesitation David replied, "Not great, actually. They say I have advanced lung cancer. I am actually in a hospital room right now. Sorry if my signal is weak; my cell phone is like five years old..."

I heard nothing else David said after that. Lung cancer? Advanced?!? He paused and I responded, "David, buddy...what can I do? Are you okay?"

He laughed his usual laugh, the one I hear so often in my mind when I think of those wonderful years we spent together growing up. "Dude, it is what it is, man! You know I've smoked since I was 15! You used to get so mad at me for smoking! Remember, I would laugh at you when you would get mad. You didn't talk to me for a week because I told you I quit, but then you busted me smoking!"

We both laughed. "I remember that!" I said, smiling to myself.

"They say it's pretty bad, buddy," David told me, sounding uncharacteristically serious. "But we both know this can't take me down. After all, I got this...I'm Batman!"

We both laughed again, and from that moment on, it was like no time had ever passed. I guess that's how it is with real friends; you can easily pick up from where you left off and 20 years can feel like 20 minutes. For the next few weeks we were like our teenage best-friend selves. We talked three times or more per day. I was traveling a lot and we lived several hours away from one another, but I knew I needed to make some time to see David, face to face. Once we found a date that worked, I bought David a Batman pillow, blanket, and t-shirt. I knew even a 50-year-old David would love them. He was still a kid at heart.

When I arrived at his hospital room, I hesitated outside the door for a minute. I felt a brief moment of fear. I hadn't seen my childhood best friend for many years, and although I didn't want to admit it, deep down I knew that his prognosis was bad. Taking a deep breath, I opened the door. As soon as I saw his face and heard his laugh—the same laugh that I remembered from back in the day—it was all good.

While David clearly looked ill, I could still see the "old David." Isn't it funny that no matter how much we age or how sick we may be, our eyes are truly those soul windows? David loved his Batman swag. We hugged and laughed and cried and hugged some more. It was awesome.

Then I went into "Rich, the Nurse" mode and wanted to know all about his care and what was going on with his treatments. He had put me on the list of people who could have access to his healthcare information, so I had a good idea of what the plan was—but I wanted to know more. "David, how are they treating you here?"

He hesitated. "Pretty good, I guess. I mean, most people are cool. I love the nurses. Well, except one. She's actually here today. Her name is Mary. I mean, she's okay. I just think that she doesn't like me. I don't know; maybe I'm being sensitive. Look, I've been upfront with everyone about my history with certain substances. But I am in a lot of pain. The tumor in my lung is wrapping around my heart and it hurts. Sometimes I just lay here with tears rolling out of my eyes. The docs tell me I should ask for pain meds whenever I need them, but whenever I ask her, she just acts weird."

I interrupted, "Weird? Like how?"

He went on, "I feel like she's judging me a little. Whenever I ask for meds, she sort of makes a face or says things like, 'Oh, more pain meds, what a surprise!' I just feel like she hates me. I don't want to complain or anything. I know how hard nurses work and all, but I am kind of scared of her, like if I bother her she won't take care of me. I don't know. Maybe I am being a baby."

As you can imagine, this really bothered me. Regardless of his past, my friend was in pain, and his medical condition warranted that he receive pain meds. At this point he was end stage and he was "scared" of a fellow nurse, lying in bed crying rather than asking for pain meds? I could feel my blood boiling. I calmed down as I didn't want to upset David. We talked a bit more and he asked me if I could run some errands for him, grab him some lunch, and let him nap for a little while.

As I walked out I noticed a nurse at a desk just outside of David's room. Her badge said "Mary." I asked if she was David's nurse, and she responded, "Can I help you with something?" I was taken aback by her tone but ignored it for a moment. I told her my name, explained that I was David's good friend, and that my name was on the list of people authorized to access his healthcare information. Mary checked and without making eye contact asked, "So, what do you need?"

I said, "How do you think he's doing?"

She paused. "Okay, considering. To be honest, he's a bit needy at times."

Keeping my cool, I responded, "Well, cancer will do that to you, won't it?"

Mary looked up and replied, "Some more than others. But if you're his friend, I am sure you know there are a few other things at play."

I assumed she meant David asking for pain meds. Her whole demeanor and tone were really getting to me, and I truly felt myself getting angry. But at that moment, I literally heard a voice in my head. The voice said, *Take another route.* I decided to "trust my gut"! So I took a breath, softened my tone, and asked, "Mary, why are you a nurse?"

This surprised her. I could tell by her face that she took my question as an aggressive challenge rather than an expression of curiosity, which was how I'd truly meant it. Mary spun toward me with a glare. She was ready for war. "Well, sir, I have been a nurse for almost five years. I am a nurse because I like to take care of people, but it is a difficult job, really difficult. It requires you to sometimes take care of people who chose not to take care of themselves. It's not easy seeing people get sick because of their own poor choices. I guess sometimes in life we get what we deserve. But that's something that only a nurse could understand. I don't expect you to get that."

I said, "Actually, I do understand. You see, Mary, I have been a nurse for almost 24 years." (I have no problem pulling seniority!) "My first job was in oncology and I can tell you why I became a nurse. It was because of my dad. My dad smoked and he got cancer, but Mary, I never saw it as a *punishment* for his choices. I saw it merely as a *consequence* of those choices. One day when I was caring for my dad, he looked up at me and said, 'You'd make a really good nurse,' and that was the moment that changed everything for me. That's why I became a nurse. Now tell me, why did *you* become a nurse?"

Mary's face completely changed. She thought for a second, lowered her eyes, and then spoke. "Actually it's very similar to your story, but it was my sister. You see, my sister and I were both raised in foster care. Sometimes that went well, sometimes not so much, but my big sister was amazing. She always looked out for me and I looked up to her. She was so talented—an amazing singer, and the funniest person I ever met. She would make me laugh so hard I'd get dizzy. Then her life kind of took some tough turns, she got into drugs and drinking, and she started smoking many packs of cigarettes a day. Then she got cancer. Our roles changed and I was taking care of her. I did it with all of my heart and it was the hardest thing I ever had to do. I hated what the drugs and smoking did to her. I hate when I see that in this world, and I see it a lot."

I could tell it was difficult for her to speak. She paused, and I said, "Mary, do you see your sister when you're taking care of David?"

She replied, "Yes…I guess I do."

"You loved a lot of things about your sister, didn't you?" I asked. Mary looked and me and nodded. I said softly, "Can you please see those qualities in my friend? You see, he was the funniest, most talented person I have ever known, he always looked out for me, and I love him like a brother. See, he's hurting, Mary, and he's really scared. He's scared of cancer, he's scared of dying, and he's scared of you. When you go back in that room, can you please see your sister?" She nodded.

We sat there quietly, us two nurses, then to my surprise Mary looked up and asked if she could hug me. She said, "I thought you were coming out here to tell me off, and when you asked me why I became a nurse I guess I took it wrong. It's just not a question you ever hear anybody asking. Why did you ask me that?"

I said, "Mary, I have learned something in my life: When you walk through a hospital or an airport or a parking garage or a hotel lobby and you see someone who clearly appears to be lost, you always have two choices. You can walk by them or you can walk over to them. It's always those two: by or over. I am not perfect, but I always try to be the guy who walks over. You seemed a little lost to me there, and I decided to walk over—that's all."

Mary asked, "So, what do you do as a nurse?" Half joking, she chuckled and added, "Do you just go around trying to inspire stressed-out healthcare people?"

I laughed. "Funny you should say that!" I told her that I speak all over North America and that I've written a couple of books. I asked her if I could send her my first book, *Inspired Nurse*. She was so appreciative, but as she was about to give me her address, she got paged overhead. She said that she'd get me her mailing information later on in her shift.

Mary started to walk away, but suddenly stopped. After standing still for about 30 or 40 seconds, she turned around, walked over to me, tilted her head quizzically, and asked, "Hey, if you don't mind my asking, what's with all of the Batman stuff you brought David? You look like you raided a toy store or something. What's that all about?"

I laughed and told her all about the childhood obsession David and I had had with Batman. I explained, "He's a fighter, Mary, and to me... that guy lying in that bed in there, he's Batman." You should've seen the look on her face. She was absolutely startled. I remember thinking to myself, *Why is she so surprised? There are lots of people who like Batman.*

Mary actually started to walk away again, but then stopped. When she turned back to me, I noticed that she was crying. Mary gingerly walked over, grabbed my arm, and in a quiet, shaky voice she whispered:

"My sister's name...was Robin."

As she walked away, leaving me stunned, I thought to myself, *Holy meant to be, Batman!* It took me a few minutes to gather my thoughts. It's amazing when things like that happen. Was it a coincidence? I doubt it. But, wow!

I left, ran some errands, and got David some lunch. By the time I returned, he had already been up for a little while and was actually hungry, which was a great thing. He looked at me with the funniest expression and said, "Dude, something happened to Mary!" I laughed and asked what he meant. He continued, "She came in here and sat with me for a while. She held my hand, she told me she was sorry if she wasn't nice before, and she shared with me that I reminded her of someone she lost. She told me that if I was ever feeling pain to let her know and she'd be on top of it. Did you say something to her?"

I nodded and told him, "Yeah, we had a little bit of a conversation."

He said, "Oh, okay, that's good. Hey, man, she told me to give you this envelope. I think she said you were sending her a book or something, and I guess it's her mailing address." Without opening it, I stuffed the envelope into my backpack.

David and I hung out for a few more hours, talking and laughing. I knew I needed to leave soon to make the long drive home, but I continued to sit on David's bed, holding his hand—just two old friends. I was trying to stay upbeat and funny, but my emotions got to me and I started to cry. Then David started to cry, and we talked honestly about all the years we'd let go by, and all the times we'd missed each other.

I apologized for being out of David's life for so long and told him that I felt I let him down. I should've been there for him when he was struggling. He laughed, pointed to his heart, and said, "You were always with me, Rich. Always." I told my friend that I loved him, and he told me I was the best friend he ever had. I guess I started getting a little too emotional so he punched my shoulder—after all, that's what friends do! Perking up and crossing his arms like a superhero, he said, "I got this, Rich…I'm Batman!" I agreed and gave David one last hug.

I remember standing in the doorway, looking at my first best friend. Lying in that bed was a 50-year-old man dying from cancer, but strangely, all I could see was my crazy, goofy, amazingly talented 14-year-old best friend smiling back at me. That's how I will always remember that moment. I slowly closed the door, walked down the hall, leaned against the wall by the elevator, and cried. The five-hour drive home was a blur. I listened to the '80s satellite radio station as moments of my youth flashed before my eyes, making me laugh and making me cry.

On May 9, 2015, at 5:48 p.m., my first best friend died peacefully. He wanted no funeral, so his beautiful sister Deanna honored his wishes to be cremated. Days later she called me and told me that she was on her way to the cremation, and that she was bringing the Batman blanket, t-shirt, and pillow that I had given David. She wanted him to have those things with him when he was cremated, she said, because "You guys were always the best of friends. He loved you so much. He was so happy that you guys reconnected. I wanted some of you to be with him forever." I will always be grateful to my little sister Deanna, the sister of my first best friend, for doing that.

I was actually sitting in the Denver airport when Deanna called me. After I hung up, I put my phone in my backpack, and as I reached into the bag I felt the envelope that David had given me in his hospital room—the one from Mary. I had forgotten all about it. When I opened the envelope, out fell a rubber Batman bracelet. Mary must've bought it in the hospital gift shop when I stepped out to run errands that day. There was a note from her that read, "I promise you I will take great care of Batman. Robin would want it no other way."

As they say, there's something about Mary, something that is within all of us in nursing: a deep connection to our *why. Why are you a nurse?* Mary reminded me that it is easy to lose that connection, in life and at work. It's a little bit like losing your GPS signal when you're driving. Without guidance, you might make a wrong turn, or two, or more.

The journeys we take often take much from us. It is an unrealistic goal, I think, to never get lost. If you've never been lost, you've probably never been on a journey. The longer and the more intense a journey is the more of a chance that you might get lost. We ALL get lost from time to time, as nurses or just as human beings.

Sometimes we lose our way because new things shake us up, make us want to pack up our "princess bag," and move out. Instead of embracing change, we throw our arms up and surrender. Sometimes we lose our way when we see injustice, when we have to deal with difficult people, when no one will listen to us even when we know what's right, or when we fail to trust our gut. Sometimes we lose our way because we forget that it is the little things that have the largest impact.

But there's often a silver lining to getting lost: It can open up doors you would've never known existed otherwise. Losing your way also brings you lessons, mentors, and friends. Remember, simply *being* lost isn't the problem; *staying* lost is. When we choose to throw our arms around the gifts and benefits that come from being lost, they will embrace us right back—and lead us back to the right path.

So, how do you reconnect with your *why* and regain your sense of direction after losing your way? Well, let's return to the GPS example.

I don't know about you, but I find that 90 percent of the time rebooting it solves whatever technological issue caused it to fail in the first place. Actually, that strategy tends to work with all of my devices, from my phone to my tablet to my laptop. After a quick restart, I can get back to work. (I say "work," but we all know I really mean Candy Crush or Angry Birds!)

Here's what I suggest the next time you need a quick "reboot" to get back to your *why*:

1. Step out of your routine. This can be as simple as reading a book, walking your dog, or going to see that movie you keep promising yourself you'll catch before it's gone from the theater. Or go to the gym. Seriously, go take a class, hit the weights, or put in some time on the elliptical—even if it's only for a few minutes. "Little" things (remember those?) like these can bring your brain and your body some distraction, laughter, or rest. Often, all it takes is a "little" (there's that word *again*!) deviation from your normal routine to help you see the path you're on with fresh eyes. Once you take a few moments to press "pause," you might just realize that for whatever reason (stress, frustration, a busy schedule, or just "going with the flow of the status quo"), you've started to lose your way and that your GPS needs recalibration.

2. Meditate. (Seriously!) EVERY super performer in business, art, or life has some type of meditative practice. I have personally listened to over 50 podcasts and watched dozens of interviews pertaining to high-performing people. One thing almost all of them had in common was that they meditated. I could write a whole book on the benefits of meditation, but there is so much out there (on the Internet, at the library, and on social media) that you don't need me to help you take that journey. I simply want to encourage you to find a technique that makes your brain happy! So take a class, get a book, watch a YouTube video, or download an app. With all of the options available, there's literally no excuse to NOT meditate…well, except for these, which I will answer since I've used them as well:

- It's too hard. (No, nursing school was hard. So really, sitting quietly is harder than your neuro clinical days as a student? Uh…I don't think so.)
- I don't have time. (Hmmm. Yes, you do. Spend a few minutes finding your center instead of watching TMZ or scrolling through Facebook…unless you're on my *Inspired Nurse* page, that is!)
- I can't shut my mind off. (Exactly! That's why you need meditation. That's like saying, "I can't take a flexibility class because I can't do a split!" The only way to improve your "mind control" is to practice it.)
- Only weird people who wear patchouli meditate. (First, patchouli smells awesome. Second, they seem weird to you only because they're not stress monsters like we are. Third, only weird people stare at total strangers' veins, fantasizing about how easy it would be to start an IV on them…so…yeah. This might be an instance of the pot calling the kettle black. Embrace the "weird"!)

So now that we have that out of the way, go sit somewhere and connect to your Spirit, God, Higher Power, or a tree you really like. Just 10 to 20 minutes a day. Get a book, app, DVD, video, or podcast on meditation. You'll be Zen before you know it!

3. Remind yourself of why nursing is incredible. Make a list of all of the things you love about being a nurse. Strive for as many as possible. Then look at each thing on the list and ask yourself, *Why do I love this?* Write a few lines, paragraphs, or pages about it. For example, let's say one thing you love is making people laugh. Take that and write a little bit about *why* you love, as part of your nursing practice, making people laugh.

I strongly suggest that you do this specific exercise with a group of nurses if you can. Write your thoughts out beforehand, then meet up, share, and discuss. (This is a great way to start or end a huddle at the beginning of a shift.) What happens here is you *all* change your focus. You're powerfully bringing to mind what you love and why you love it. I don't want to spoil the surprise, but I do want to tell you that if you do this, alone or with a group, you may be truly amazed at how much your attitude changes and at how (re)inspired you become!

Here's the bottom line: Being a nurse is an incredible journey. And if you think about it, you'll realize that you are never the same after a journey. Hopefully the person you are right now is not the same person you were when you first picked up this book. Please know that the journey to inspiration is a very deep and personal one. You travel down that road every day with every patient you take care of, every coworker you help, and every new nurse you teach.

I know that sometimes it gets hard to continue moving forward—really, really hard. And it's because you care. If you didn't care, you wouldn't be reading this book. So if you ever doubt yourself, even a little, or if you ever wonder, *How can I do this any longer?* please just remember:

You got this…you're Batman!

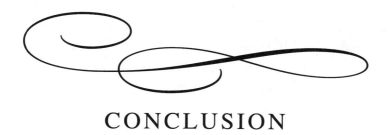

CONCLUSION

You've made it! This is the end of the book! So...do you feel more inspired? Did you see yourself in some of these stories, or did you maybe recall something similar that happened to you? I hope so. We are part of a remarkable family, aren't we? Nurses are truly the most amazing people on earth. We do incredible things—miraculous things—every day. Fueled by passion, skill, love, intellect, spirit...and coffee...nurses rock!

Because nurses *do* rock and *are* so amazing, I have a few final requests I'd like to make of you.

First, when you *are* feeling inspired, when you're having one of those days when you are rocking, look around you. If you see one of your nurse peers struggling, feeling uninspired, having a bad day, or showing signs of burn-out, please reach out with an encouraging word or a listening ear. Maybe even lend them this book or buy them one of their own. We need to help each other. Only a nurse understands what another nurse deals with. If I may borrow a line from our heroic service men and women...Leave no nurse behind.

Second, please be kind to yourself—*especially* when you're struggling to feel inspired. With all you give to others, please show a little generosity to yourself. With all you do for others, please also do for yourself. With all the time, energy, and passion you put into healing others, can you find some time, energy, and passion to heal yourself? This world needs you. Yes, you!

Bearing that in mind, allow me to add another thought—maybe one of the most important of all. If you are truly struggling beyond the scope of what I've shared here; if you're dealing with depression or anxiety or addiction; or if you're just in deep doubt or pain about nursing, life, or whatever, please don't hesitate to seek out professional help. Our fellow healthcare workers in the mental/behavioral health world are amazing. A good therapist or practitioner could make an amazing difference in your life. Please?

I'm not a huge fan of goodbyes. So I'll end this book by saying that I hope you feel different now from when you started reading—and I hope it shows. If anyone looks at you over the next few days and notices that you're smiling a little more and stressing a little less, maybe they'll say to you, "What are you doing? You seem different."

Share with them what you've learned. Maybe there was one story or example in these pages that really popped for you. If so, please pass it on! I wrote this book because I want you to be an Inspired Nurse...so help the next nurse be an Inspired Nurse Too!

Thank you for what you do for your patients, teams, peers, profession...and the world. You are a light in the darkness. You are a gift and a blessing. You are what the world needs.

So go out there and be that amazing, daring, beautiful, brilliant, heroic, and inspired nurse that you are.

Never doubt for one minute the amazingness that is YOU.

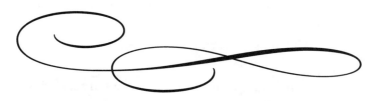

ACKNOWLEDGMENTS

I would like to gratefully acknowledge and thank the following, in no specific order, but with very specific love and affection:

Bekki Kennedy, for your dedication, friendship, and always believing. This book wouldn't have happened without you.

B.G. Porter, for being a mentor when you didn't have to be and a friend because you wanted to be. I'm so grateful for all you've done.

Liz Jazwiec, for making me laugh and making me think. You're a beautiful soul and a true friend.

Lindy Sikes, for your heart and for sending me Batman emails.

Jamie Stewart, for your focus, hard work, and friendship.

Dan Collard, for being my brother and friend. Always.

Renee Barnett, Melanie Carpenter, Genevieve Kurpuis, and Dee Dee Thompkins. Your support and friendship are as priceless as your beautiful spirits. Thanks for caring about me.

Stephen Dickerson. You're brilliant and I'm blessed to work with you.

Stephanie Barbee, Sara Harris, Laura Koontz, Tasha Wells, and Lauren Westwood, for your friendship and all you do to make me look so much better than I could ever do on my own.

Matthew Bates, Brad Braddock, Don Dean, George Ellis, Debbie Ritchie, and the Studer Group senior leaders, I'm grateful to work with you, learn from you, and, mostly, to call you friends.

Craig Deao. I'm appreciative of your support and so fortunate to work with you.

Bob Murphy, for making work fun for me whenever I see you.

Dottie DeHart and team. You're always rock stars.

All of Studer Group. Each of you makes healthcare better. You are my family, and I love you all.

My mom, Ann, your love and wisdom are a blessing to me. I hit the lottery getting you as my mother.

My brothers, Jack and Bob. Thanks for all you've done for me. I love you both so much.

Acknowledgments

My mother-in-law, Vickie. You are an incredible person with a huge heart. Thank you for everything.

Julie Bluni, you are so special to me. Thanks for loving Dawn and me and our kids. We love you right back.

Art, Fonda, Rowen, and Ella. Thanks for loving us.

Jason, Tyler, and Kloe. You are my family, and I love you more than words can express.

Karen and Tom. I'm so lucky to have you as friends.

Tony, Angela, and Nicholas. You are so special to me. I love you guys.

Al, Gina, and Nevin. Grateful for your friendship and love. Collunis forever!

John F. Kennedy and Jackie. Living next to the Kennedy compound is a blessing to my family. Love you guys.

Shane, Michelle, and Tanner. Thank you for always being there for my family and me. You're amazing friends. Your family is my family. Our pasta is your pasta.

Sam, Scott, Lila, and Gunner. I'm so lucky to have you in my life. We love you guys so much. No one throws better dance parties.

Al, Jeannie, and their amazing family. So many years of laughter and smiles. You mean the world to me.

Peter, Jennifer, PJ, and Olivia. We love you pineapples!

Jennifer Rose Allen. Thanks for being there for our family. You are very special to us.

David Zambrana. I love you, brother!

Deanna Hernandez. I am grateful for all you did for David and for allowing me to be there. You're the best sister ever.

Quint Studer. What you started will never end. The good you've done will last forever. I'm so lucky to call you my friend.

To nurses everywhere. You are the most amazing human beings. You give so much. The world is a better place because of you. I love each of you, my sisters and brothers.

My Inspired Nurse Facebook peeps. I'm honored and grateful that you support me.

Rhett, you make me so proud. I love you, son.

Luke, you fill my heart. I love you, son.

Ava, you make me smile. I love you, princess.

Dawn, I love you from the top of Heaven and back.

To my dad, Jack. Thanks for watching over me.

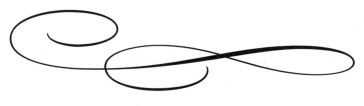

ADDITIONAL RESOURCES

ABOUT STUDER GROUP®, A HURON HEALTHCARE SOLUTION:

Learn more about Studer Group® by scanning the QR code with your mobile device or by visiting www.studergroup.com/who-we-are/about-studer-group.

A recipient of the 2010 Malcolm Baldrige National Quality Award, Studer Group is an outcomes-based healthcare performance improvement firm that works with healthcare organizations in the United States, Canada, and beyond, teaching them how to achieve, sustain, and accelerate exceptional clinical, operational, and financial results. Working together, we help to get the foundation right so organizations can build a sustainable culture that promotes accountability, fosters innovation, and consistently delivers a great patient experience and the best quality outcomes over time.

To learn more about Studer Group, a Huron Healthcare solution, visit www.studergroup.com or call 850-439-5839.

STUDER GROUP COACHING:
Learn more about Studer Group coaching by scanning the QR code with your mobile device or by visiting www.studergroup.com/coaching.

Studer Group coaches partner with healthcare organizations to create an aligned culture accountable to achieving outcomes together. Working side-by-side, we help to establish, accelerate, and hardwire the necessary changes to create a culture of excellence. This leads to better transparency, higher accountability, and the ability to target and execute specific, objective results that organizations want to achieve.

Studer Group offers coaching based on organizational needs: Evidence-Based Leadership, System Partnership, Specialized Emergency Department, Huron Physician Solutions, Medical Practice, and Rural Healthcare.

BOOKS: CATEGORIZED BY AUDIENCE

Explore the Fire Starter Publishing website by scanning the QR code with your mobile device or by visiting www.firestarterpublishing.com.

<u>Senior Leaders & Physicians</u>

A Culture of High Performance: Achieving Higher Quality at a Lower Cost—A must-have book for any leader struggling to shore up margins while sustaining an organization that is a great place for employees to work, physicians to practice medicine, and patients to receive care. From best-selling author Quint Studer to help you build a culture that will thrive during change.

Straight A Leadership: Alignment, Action, Accountability—A guide that will help you identify gaps in alignment, action, and accountability; create a plan to fill them; and become a more resourceful, agile, high-performing organization, written by Quint Studer.

Engaging Physicians: A Manual to Physician Partnership—A tactical and passionate road map for physician collaboration to generate organizational high performance, written by Stephen C. Beeson, MD.

Excellence with an Edge: Practicing Medicine in a Competitive Environment—An insightful book that provides practical tools and techniques you need to know to have a solid grasp of the business side of making a living in healthcare, written by Michael T. Harris, MD.

Physicians

Healing Physician Burnout: Diagnosing, Preventing, and Treating—
Written by Quint Studer, in collaboration with George Ford, MD,
this book helps leaders and physicians work together to create healthy
environments for practicing medicine while navigating the huge
changes disrupting our industry. It explores why physicians are so
burned out and provides practical tools to get them engaged, aligned,
and reconnected to their sense of meaning and purpose.

*The CG CAHPS Handbook: A Guide to Improve Patient Experience and
Clinical Outcomes*—Written by Jeff Morris, MD, MBA, FACS; Bar-
bara Hotko, RN, MPA; and Matthew Bates, MPH. *The CG CAHPS
Handbook* is your guide for consistently delivering on what matters
most to patients and their families and for providing exceptional care
and improved clinical outcomes.

*Practicing Excellence: A Physician's Manual to Exceptional Health
Care*—This book, written by Stephen C. Beeson, MD, is a brilliant
guide to implementing physician leadership and behaviors that will
create a high-performance workplace.

All Leaders

101 Answers to Questions Leaders Ask—By Quint Studer and Studer
Group coaches, offers practical, prescriptive solutions from healthcare
leaders around the country.

*Eat That Cookie!: Make Workplace Positivity Pay Off...For Individuals,
Teams, and Organizations*—Written by Liz Jazwiec, RN, this book is

funny, inspiring, relatable, and is packed with realistic, down-to-earth tactics to infuse positivity into your culture.

Hardwiring Excellence—A *BusinessWeek* bestseller, this book is a road map to creating and sustaining a "Culture of Service and Operational Excellence" that drives bottom-line results. Written by Quint Studer.

Hey Cupcake! We Are ALL Leaders—Author Liz Jazwiec explains that we'll all eventually be called on to lead someone, whether it's a department, a shift, a project team, or a new employee. In her trademark slightly sarcastic (and hilarious) voice, she provides learned-the-hard-way insights that will benefit leaders in every industry and at every level.

"I'm Sorry to Hear That..." Real-Life Responses to Patients' 101 Most Common Complaints About Health Care—When you respond to a patient's complaint, you are responding to the patient's sense of helplessness and anxiety. The service recovery scripts offered in this book can help you recover a patient's confidence in you and your organization. Authored by Susan Keane Baker and Leslie Bank.

Oh No...Not More of That Fluffy Stuff! The Power of Engagement— Written by Rich Bluni, RN, this funny, heartfelt book explores what it takes to overcome obstacles and tap into the passion that fuels our best work. Its practical exercises help employees at all levels get happier, more excited, and more connected to the meaning in our daily lives.

Over Our Heads: An Analogy on Healthcare, Good Intentions, and Unforeseen Consequences— This book, written by Rulon F. Stacey, PhD,

FACHE, uses a grocery store analogy to illustrate how government intervention leads to economic crisis and, eventually, collapse.

Results That Last: Hardwiring Behaviors That Will Take Your Company to the Top—A *Wall Street Journal* bestseller by Quint Studer that teaches leaders in every industry how to apply his tactics and strategies to their own organizations to build a corporate culture that consistently reaches and exceeds its goals.

Service Excellence Is As Easy As PIE (Perception Is Everything)—Realistic, down to earth, and wickedly witty, *PIE* is perfect for everyone in healthcare or any other service industry. It's filled with ideas for creating exceptional customer experiences—ideas that are surprising, simple, and yes, easy as you-know-what. Written by Liz Jazwiec.

Taking Conversations from Difficult to Doable—Have you ever dreaded holding a tough but necessary conversation with an employee, co-worker, or boss? This book helps you "bite the bullet" and say what needs saying. Learn tools and tactics to navigate tough conversations confidently and effectively. Written by Lynne Cunningham.

The Great Employee Handbook: Making Work and Life Better—This book is a valuable resource for employees at all levels who want to learn how to handle tough workplace situations—skills that normally come only from a lifetime of experience. *Wall Street Journal* best-selling author Quint Studer has pulled together the best insights gained from working with thousands of employees during his career.

Wait a Hot Minute!: How to Manage Life with the Minutes You Have—When did perpetual distraction and multi-tasking become the new normal? This book helps you get real about all the ways you're squandering your most precious resource and lays out some practical tips to help you refocus on the things that really matter. Written by Jacquelyn Gaines.

Nurse Leaders and Nurses

Inspired Nurse and *Inspired Journal*—By Rich Bluni, RN, help maintain and recapture the inspiration nurses felt at the start of their journey with action-oriented "spiritual stretches" and stories that illuminate those sacred moments we all experience.

The HCAHPS Handbook, 2nd Edition: Tactics to Improve Quality and the Patient Experience—Revised and released in 2015, this book is a valuable resource for organizations seeking to provide the exceptional quality of care their patients expect and deserve. Coauthored by Lyn Ketelsen, RN, MBA; Karen Cook, RN; and Bekki Kennedy.

The Nurse Leader Handbook: The Art and Science of Nurse Leadership—By Studer Group senior nursing and physician leaders from across the country, is filled with knowledge that provides nurse leaders with a solid foundation for success. It also serves as a reference they can revisit again and again when they have questions or need a quick refresher course in a particular area of the job.

Emergency Department Team

Advance Your Emergency Department: Leading in a New Era—As this critical book asserts, world-class Emergency Departments don't follow. They lead. Stephanie J. Baker, RN, CEN, MBA; Regina Shupe, RN, MSN, CEN; and Dan Smith, MD, FACEP, share high-impact strategies and tactics to help your ED get results more efficiently, effectively, and collaboratively. Master them and you'll improve quality, exceed patient expectations, and ultimately help the entire organization maintain and grow its profit margin.

Excellence in the Emergency Department: How to Get Results—A book by Stephanie Baker, RN, CEN, MBA, is filled with proven, easy-to-implement, step-by-step instructions that will help you move your Emergency Department forward.

Hardwiring Flow: Systems and Processes for Seamless Patient Care—Drs. Thom Mayer and Kirk Jensen delve into one of the most critical issues facing healthcare leaders: patient flow.

The Patient Flow Advantage: How Hardwiring Hospital-Wide Flow Drives Competitive Performance—Build effectiveness, efficiency, and a patient-centric focus into the heart of every process that serves the patient. Efficient patient flow has never been more critical to ensure patient safety, satisfaction, and optimal reimbursement. Authored by Drs. Kirk Jensen and Thom Mayer.

STUDER CONFERENCES:
Learn more about Studer Group conferences by scanning the QR code with your mobile device or by visiting www.studergroup.com/conferences.

Studer Conferences are three-day interactive learning events designed to provide healthcare leaders with an authentic, practical learning experience. Each Studer Conference includes internationally renowned keynote speakers and tracks concentrated on key areas of the healthcare organization. Every track includes breakout sessions and "how-to" workshops that provide you with direct access to experts and conference faculty. The faculty at Studer Conferences go beyond PowerPoint slides and lectures to show you "what right looks like."

Leaders will leave with new tools and skills that get results. Find out more about upcoming Studer Conferences and register at www.studergroup.com/conferences.

All Studer Group Conferences offer Continuing Education Credits. For more information on CMEs, visit www.studergroup.com/cme-credits.

STUDER SPEAKING:
Learn more about Studer Group speaking by scanning the QR code with your mobile device or by visiting www.studergroup.com/speaking.

From large association events to exclusive executive training, Studer Group speakers deliver the perfect balance of inspiration and education for every audience. As experienced clinicians and administrators, each speaker has a unique journey to share. This personal touch along with hard-hitting healthcare improvement tactics empower your team to take action and drive organizational growth with training that reaches leaders at all levels.

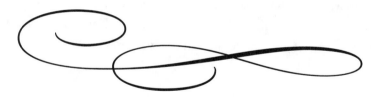

ABOUT THE AUTHOR

A force in healthcare cultural excellence, Rich Bluni, RN, is a wildly popular speaker and author. His award-winning first book, *Inspired Nurse*, has been read and loved by nurses across the globe, followed by *Oh No…Not More of That Fluffy Stuff!*, which put employee engagement on the to-do list of healthcare executives. Using social media as a platform to communicate with his followers and fans, his #MyInspiredSign challenge went viral and is still actively participated in by healthcare professionals.

Rich joined Studer Group® in 2007 as an expert coach working with organizations all over the U.S. A Registered Nurse and Licensed Healthcare Risk Manager, his clinical experience includes over 24 years in Pediatric Oncology, Pediatric Intensive Care, Flight Nursing, Trauma Intensive Care, Quality and Risk Management, and Emergency Department Leadership. He is one of Studer Group's most sought-after keynote speakers for major healthcare conferences and has presented to tens of thousands of healthcare leaders, executives, and frontline staff at hundreds of healthcare organizations, hospitals, and medical practices in the United States and Canada.

Rich is married to the love of his life, Dawn, who is also a Registered Nurse, and has two sons and a daughter, Rhett, Luke, and Ava, who keep him inspired and make him smile every day.

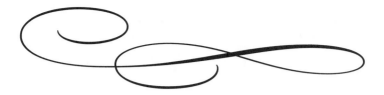

LET'S STAY IN TOUCH!

This isn't the end of your journey to inspiration…and hopefully it isn't the end of our connection, either!

I'd love to come out and speak at your conference or hospital, or you can see me speak at my organization's awesome Studer Conferences. You can find more information about where I'm speaking and how to bring me to your organization at www.studergroup.com/people/rich-bluni.

I also have a Facebook page called Inspired Nurse where I regularly post my musings on healthcare, upcoming events, and chat with an active community of nurses and other healthcare professionals. Come join us!

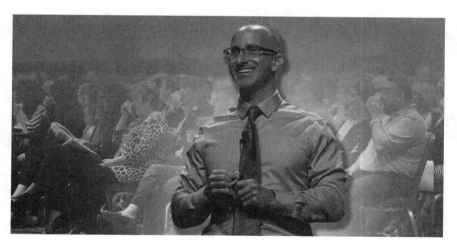

 Inspired Nurse   @InspiredNurse   InspiredNurseRichBluni

HOW TO ORDER ADDITIONAL COPIES OF

Inspired Nurse Too

Orders may be placed:

Online at:
www.firestarterpublishing.com/inspired-nurse-too

Scan the QR code with your mobile device to order through the Fire Starter
Publishing website.

By phone at: 866-354-3473

By mail at: Fire Starter Publishing
350 W. Cedar Street, Suite 300
Pensacola, FL 32502

Share this book with your team—and save!
Inspired Nurse Too is filled with inspirational and practical information.
If purchasing for a team to share, please contact Fire Starter Publishing at
866-354-3473 to learn more about volume savings.